CLAIRE MARTIN

The Nursing Mother's Problem Solver

A FIRESIDE BOOK
Published by Simon & Schuster
NEW YORK LONDON TORONTO SYDNEY SINGAPORE

FIRESIDE
Rockefeller Center
1230 Avenue of the Americas
New York, NY 10020

This publication contains the opinions and ideas of its authors and is designed to provide useful advice in regard to the subject matter covered. Statements made by the authors regarding certain products, services, and organizations are based on the authors' research, and do not constitute an endorsement of any product, service, or organization by the authors or publisher, each of whom specifically disclaims any responsibility for any liability, loss or risk, personal or otherwise, which is incurred as a consequence, directly or indirectly, of the use and application of any of the contents of this book or any of the products, services, or organizations mentioned herein. The authors urge all nursing mothers to check with your physician before taking any over-the-counter drug, herbal remedy, or vitamin supplement, and to inform the doctor prescribing medications for you that you are breastfeeding.

Designed by Songhee Kim

Manufactured in the United States of America

10 9 8 7 6 5 4 3 2 1

Library of Congress Cataloging-in-Publication Data
Martin, Claire.
The nursing mother's problem solver / Claire Martin.
p. cm.
Includes index.
1. Breast feeding—Popular works. I. Title.

RJ216.M335 2000
649'.33—dc21 00-037198

ISBN 0-684-85784-7

Acknowledgments

My agent, Jody Rein, whose tireless advocacy for this book was both personal and professional; Dr. William Sears and his wife, Martha; Carol Brussel, IBCLC, who contributed many hours of advice and exemplary editing; the Mother's Milk Bank at Presbyterian–St. Luke's Hospital in Denver; Kelly Kittel; pediatric nurse practitioner Pat Sheans; Cody Martin; ILCA representative Terry Shell; pediatrician Dr. Jack Newman; Beth Gabrielski, lactation consultant at Denver Children's Hospital; Erick Kirshner of the Colorado Foundation for Medical Care; Jenny Deam; Mary Louise Butler; Marianne "Dr. Mom" Neifert; the regular posters on alt.support.breastfeeding and misc.kids.breastfeeding; models Veronica Vasquez and Carolyn Wiese; Usenet breastfeeding gurus Angela Beegle and Larry McMahan; Trish Todd, my thorough and resourceful editor at Simon & Schuster; Diane Carman, Howard Saltz, and other supportive editors and colleagues at *The Denver Post*; my daughters, Cordelia and Tessa, who taught me firsthand the problems and joys of breastfeeding; and my patient husband, Bruce Finley, without whose love, support, and patience this book would not exist.

For my mother

Foreword

There are plenty of books that explain why you should breastfeed, and can teach you the basics, but this is the first designed specifically as a panic button for harried new mothers.

Whether you're a first-time mother or a veteran mom, the first few weeks of a baby's life are stressful and pressured. That's where this new and different breastfeeding guide fits in. It focuses on the questions that often come up at midnight or 2 A.M., when you're hesitant to call your doctor or lactation consultant and you know it will be hours before you'll be able to call your health care provider's help line.

This book covers the most common problems and issues associated with breastfeeding, and offers tips on how to solve those problems or alleviate them until you can get medical attention.

Most important, this book is written by mothers who have been in your shoes. Claire Martin and Nancy Krebs know how tempting it is to join a frustrated, screaming baby in a duet. They've survived erratic sleeping jags and the marathon nursing sessions of growth spurts. They are the friends you can trust and turn to for reliable advice that comes from hard-won experience.

Think of *The Nursing Mother's Problem Solver* as your first-defense reference book for breastfeeding questions — a supplement to your parenting library. Open this book when you need a quick answer or helpful advice. This book won't answer all your questions — no book can — and certainly is not a substitute for your doctor or lactation consultant. But if, between visits and phone calls, a worrisome symptom appears, or if you've forgotten a step in settling your baby in a comfortable nursing position, you'll be glad you keep this book handy.

William and Martha Sears
Authors of *The Breastfeeding Book*

Preface

In paintings and photographs, nursing mothers look so serene, and the babies so docile, that most of us just assume that breastfeeding is natural and easy. Then it's your turn to be the nursing mom in the picture, and suddenly breastfeeding is about as easy and natural as flying solo. There's a big difference between "natural" and "easy." (Is "natural childbirth" easy? Not for most of us.)

Nanoseconds after she was born, my first child lay between my desperately engorged breasts and looked at me with an expression of introspective bewilderment: Now what? That pretty much summed up my feelings. Her head was smaller than my swollen right breast. How was I supposed to get my nipple, and the vast sea of areola surrounding it, into that tiny red mouth?

"Uh, uh, uh," she said, her mouth yearning toward a nipple.

Eventually we figured it out. Breastfeeding has a heck of a learning curve. Almost every woman who breastfeeds her baby runs into problems at some point. Some of us are lucky initially — our babies latch on like champs after delivery — but then we get a yeast infection or a plugged duct, or discover that the baby who nursed so beautifully yesterday absolutely refuses to latch on today. (Or we discover that the baby wants to nurse every 30 minutes.) It takes a while to figure out whether the baby is eating to satiation or latching on well, and to tell the difference between a baby who eats frequently because she's getting only foremilk, and a baby who eats frequently because she's going through a growth spurt.

And then, once you think you've figured it all out, you wake up with the dizzying fever that signals mastitis. Or you get thrush. Or the baby is teething and (a) wants to nurse constantly, especially when a disapproving in-law is watching, or (b) pushes your watermelon-tight breast away, ignoring the milk that sprays in his face. Or you need to rent or buy a breast pump that poses an entirely new set of questions. These are the reasons for this book. It's meant to help you identify and begin solving problems. Just as *Cliff's Notes* provide a shortcut to the themes in classic literature, this is *Cliff's Notes* for breastfeeding moms. All the questions in this book are real, and so are the nursing moms who asked them — sometimes when they were on the brink of giving up. Their questions came from interviews with new nursing mothers, from questions called in to pediatricians and lactation consultants, and from questions posted on online newsgroups organized by breastfeeding mothers, pediatricians, and lactation consultants. When you're wondering whether your symptoms indicate thrush or an inflamed breast, or whether it's okay to have a beer just once instead of another glass of iced tea; when nothing seems to help your cracked nipples, or if you're having trouble getting a tiny newborn mouth to latch onto a nipple the size of his face, turn to this book. You'll find answers and suggestions.

And, of course, you'll learn a lot of things on your own. For instance:

- When you're breastfeeding, you tell time by considering how long it's been since the last feeding. (And even that goes out the window when the baby is sick, is teething, or is going through a growth spurt.)
- When you're breastfeeding, you choose clothing according to how easily your breasts can be accessed. (This pretty much rules out tank dresses, jumpers, and one-piece outfits.) You choose fabrics with an eye for a pattern that camouflages leaking milk and spit-up. Silk is out. Dark is out. You learn to see vests as utilitarian wardrobe staples rather than cute but optional accessories.
- When you're breastfeeding, you learn to drink more than a marathon runner. (In fact, having little cups of water and juice set up at intervals along your daily route strikes you as a pretty good idea.)

- When you're breastfeeding, "the wet spot" in your bed is the part of the sheet directly under your chest. A lot of nursing moms resign themselves to wearing a bra 24 hours a day — with nursing pads.
- And when you're breastfeeding, you discover a new level of blissed-out love. There is no feeling on earth like locking eyes with a baby who is peacefully nursing at your breast. It is a peace that the most beatific madonna-and-child painting falls short of depicting.

This is the way breastfeeding is supposed to be. And it is easy. And it does feel natural.

How to Use This Book

The Nursing Mother's Problem Solver is designed to be a sort of breastfeeding thesaurus—a resource you can count on when you need a swift answer that can be easily found, even when it's 3 A.M. and you're at the end of your rope, with a squalling baby in one hand and this book in the other.

The wealth of material that follows is alphabetically organized to help you quickly find the specific topic you're seeking. It also includes cross-references that direct you to additional information on the same topic or related issues.

For example, if you're concerned about a red, painfully tender place on your breast, you can go to "Red Streak" in the "R" section for an in-depth explanation that also refers you to entries on plugged ducts and mastitis, two conditions that may be related. Or, if you're struggling with a frantic baby, you can look up "Frantic Nurser" to find an answer that also directs you to entries on breast compression, colic, growth spurts, and overactive letdown — techniques and situations that can help you better understand your baby, and resolve the situation.

You'll find the answers to common problems — getting the baby to latch on, growth spurts that go hand in hand with nonstop nursing, how to stock your nursing station, the merits of gliders versus rocking chairs, and more — that vex most new mothers. You'll also find information that most other breastfeeding books don't address, including schedule feeding programs, whether nipple jewelry affects breastfeeding, and whether exposure to tear gas can compromise your breast milk.

It won't be long before you're an expert at breastfeeding. Enjoy this special time with your baby!

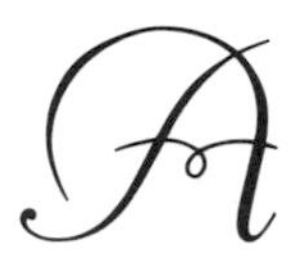

Abscess, Breast

Q: I was just diagnosed with a breast abscess, the result of a plugged duct on my right breast. My obstetrician put me on antibiotics and told me to nurse on that breast first. I finally had to have surgery to drain the abscess. The incision seems to be healing, but my milk supply in the affected breast has diminished. Will I be able to make enough milk again to continue exclusively breastfeeding my 3-month-old? Could the abscess come back?

A: If you continue nursing, your supply should gradually increase, although it may not be as high as it once was. Breast abscesses are nasty, and they can become reinfected, especially if surgery fails to drain all the pus.

You'll need to take special care if you're prone to plugged ducts. Massage your breasts when you're nursing or pumping, to loosen any plugs starting to form. Use warm compresses on your breasts just before a nursing session.

To increase your supply, drink lots of water, and get some help so you can rest up. You'll need a recovery period while your milk supply rebuilds as you recover from the abscess. Your spouse and/or other relatives and friends can do the chores while you and the baby loll in bed, napping and nursing. Drink plenty of water and juice to stay well hydrated. (If your urine is clear, or nearly clear, you're drinking enough fluids. If it's yellow, you're dehydrated.)

See also Mastitis, About; Plugged Ducts, About

Adopted Baby

Q: I'm adopting a 5-month-old baby soon, and currently I'm breastfeeding my 20-month-old. Do you have any tips on getting a 5-month-old interested in breastfeeding again? She's been bottle-fed all her life.

A: Since you're already lactating, you don't need to worry about how much milk you're producing. Other nonlactating adoptive moms who want to breastfeed must work through the slow process of inducing lactation, which can take weeks or months. With persistence and patience, and help from a breast pump, it's possible to lactate even if you've never nursed a baby.

However, it's impossible to predict how much milk you'll be able to produce on top of your current supply. You will need to increase your milk supply, since a 5-month-old nurses more than a 20-month-old whose calories also come from solids. Even then, you may not be able to exclusively breastfeed the new baby.

Expect nipple confusion problems, along with bewilderment from your new baby, who'll be wondering what the heck you're doing. Bottle-fed babies may be used to eating as they're held upright and facing away from you. Teaching them to nurse goes against everything they associate with food, and the first attempts may be upsetting for both of you.

You can try a transition using a tube feeding lactation aid—with surgical tubing taped to your breasts and nipples—so the baby connects nipples with food. Nipple shields are another option. Some adoptive moms have used a combination of both, threading the supplemental tube through an enlarged hole in the nipple shield.

There are some books about adoptive breastfeeding. Go online and check out www2.promom.org and its bookstore. There's also a Web site devoted to the issue at www.prismnet.com~naomi/abrw/. La Leche League International has archives with other stories from adoptive mothers who nursed.

See also Nipple Confusion; Nipple Shields; Tube Feeding Lactation Aids

Alcohol and Breastfeeding, About

Can a nursing mother have a glass of wine with dinner, or will the alcohol affect the baby? Should you believe your grandmother's advice to drink a beer or two in the afternoon to boost your evening milk supply? Should you pump and dump after having a margarita?

First, the bad news: The alcohol you drink does show up in your breast milk.

The good news: The percentage of alcohol in your breast milk is comparable with your blood alcohol level, not the proof on the bottle. We're talking about alcohol-flavored breast milk, not giving your infant a straight shot of whisky. A 120-pound woman would have to drink 350 5-ounce glasses of wine before her milk contained as much alcohol as the wine in her glass—a feat as improbable as it is lethal.

Here's a more realistic scenario: If a 120-pound woman has a 5-ounce glass of wine (about 12 percent alcohol), her blood alcohol level will be about 0.03 percent. Every 20 to 30 minutes after she finishes the glass of wine, the alcohol level in her blood—and therefore in her milk—diminishes by half as the liver metabolizes the alcohol.

But every individual responds differently to alcohol. Your reaction to an alcoholic drink depends on your age, your weight, your physical condition, how long it takes you to finish a drink, and the amount of food and other drugs or medications you've consumed. As a rule, the less you weigh, the more swiftly your blood alcohol percentage will rise. Two drinks will put a 140-pound woman's blood alcohol percentage at 0.07 percent (enough to significantly affect her driving ability), but it would take three drinks to elevate a 200-pound woman's blood alcohol level to the same percentage. And you'd feel fairly tipsy at 0.07 percent—in most states, a blood alcohol level of 0.08 percent is defined as the legal limit for driving under the influence.

If you follow the strict definition of moderate drinking—no more than one drink a day—it is not necessary to pump and dump afterward. Pumping will not hasten the elimination of the alcohol-flavored milk. Only time will reduce the level of alcohol in your body. If you do drink beyond the point of tipsiness and your breasts are engorged, the conservative recommendation is to pump and dump your milk instead of nursing while you're still inebriated. (If your baby is hungry before you're sober, give her some previously expressed milk.) Watching that hard-won milk go down the drain is painful enough to discourage most of us from going on a bender.

Alcohol will have an effect on your baby, according to an American Academy of Pediatrics study. Generally, babies react to alcohol-flavored milk by being more wakeful, instead of sedated, and they may be more irritable than usual.

Bear in mind that an infant—with a body weight of 10 to 20 pounds and immature organs—is far more sensitive to even small amounts of alcohol than you are, especially if she's exclusively breastfed. Studies by the American Academy of Pediatrics have shown a small but distinct relationship between maternal alcohol use and infant sleep patterns. One study demonstrated a link between maternal drinking and decreased motor skills in the infant. (Go to http://nursingbaby.com/quest6.htm for links to medical research citations.)

In short, the effect of alcohol-flavored breast milk on a baby seems to be related to the amount of alcohol that the mother drinks.

It ought to go without saying that routine abuse of alcohol will interfere with your ability to care for your baby, and it can screw up your supply and letdown, not to mention your baby's motor development, sleep patterns, and weight gain. In other words: If you drink to excess, use formula instead.

Still, breast milk from a mom who has only a glass of wine or beer a day is nutritionally better for your baby than formula. If you choose to drink in moderation, it would be a good idea to wait until your infant has fallen asleep (for one of her longer naps) or to limit your alcohol use to special occasions.

See also Pumping, About

Alcohol, Effect on Breast Milk

Q: I know that some alcohol from a drink probably leaches into breast milk. But if I have one glass of wine, or one beer, will the amount of alcohol that makes it into the breast milk harm my 1-month-old daughter? I'm not talking about getting drunk—just having a beer or a glass of wine a few times a week.

A: Alcohol does leach into your breast milk—it can be detected in breast milk about 30 minutes after you have a drink (12 ounces of beer, 5 ounces of wine, or 1.25 ounces of 80-proof liquor). Most physicians and lactation consultants in the United States advise breastfeeding moms to lay off the hooch. Some pediatricians and lactation consultants say that a glass of wine or a bottle of beer, even once a day, is fine as long as you don't drink to the point of feeling high or drunk. One or two beers (12 ounces apiece) or a glass of wine (5 ounces) each week won't harm your baby.

As you'd expect, the effect that alcohol-infused breast milk has on a baby is directly related to the amount that the mother drinks. Think of it this way: The amount of alcohol that leaches into your milk is equivalent to your blood alcohol level. If you've had enough alcohol to impair your driving ability (see the BAC Chart for Women), you've had enough to affect your baby.

Alcohol does have an effect on babies. It screws up their sleeping schedule and makes them more wakeful and more fretful, according to a recent study published by the American Academy of Pediatrics. (That prospect is enough to make juice or soda far more appealing than a beer.) Babies whose mothers drink two or more alcoholic beverages a day—a level that exceeds "moderate" drinking as defined by the National Clearinghouse for Alcohol and Drug Information—do show measurable developmental delays. Some lactation consultants advise nursing moms to avoid nursing for up to 3 hours after having a drink. Others say that you don't need to refrain from nursing unless you feel the effects of a drink, and one drink shouldn't do that. Your best bet: If you want a beer or a glass of wine, try to nurse the baby just before you have the drink.

See also Alcohol and Breastfeeding, About

BAC CHART FOR WOMEN

Correlate number of drinks to body weight to find approximate blood alcohol concentration (percentage, expressed as decimal value). Values in boldface indicate significant impairment of skills

Body Weight in Pounds

Number of Drinks	90	100	120	140	160	180	200	220	240	
0	.00	.00	.00	.00	.00	.00	.00	.00	.00	Only safe driving limit
1	05	.05	.04	.03	.03	.03	.02	.02	.02	Impairment begins
2	**.10**	.09	.08	.07	.06	.05	.05	.04	.04	Driving skills significantly affected; possible criminal penalties
3	**.15**	**.14**	**.11**	**.10**	.09	.08	.07	.06.	06	
4	**.20**	**.18**	**.15**	**.13**	**.11**	**.10**	**.09**	.08	.08	
5	**.25**	**.23**	**.19**	**.16**	**.14**	**.13**	**.11**	**.10**	.09	
6	**.30**	**.27**	**.23**	**.19**	**.17**	**.15**	**.14**	**.12**	**.11**	Legally intoxicated; criminal penalties
7	**.35**	**.32**	**.27**	**.23**	**.20**	**.18**	**.16**	**.14**	**.13**	
8	**.40**	**.36**	**.30**	**.26**	**.23**	**.20**	**.18**	**.17**	**.15**	
9	**.45**	**.41**	**.34**	**.29**	**.26**	**.23**	**.20**	**.19**	**.17**	
10	**.51**	**.45**	**.38**	**.32**	**.28**	**.25**	**.23**	**.21**	**.19**	

Subtract .01% for each 40 minutes of drinking.
One drink is 1.25 oz. of 80 proof liquor, 12 oz. of beer, or 5 oz. of table wine.

Source: Be Responsible About Drinking, Inc. (B.R.A.D.). See Web site at <http://www.brad21.org/bac_charts.html>.

Allergies (Baby's), About

If you're sensitive to certain foods, your baby may be, too. Babies are more likely to be sensitive to certain foods rather than truly allergic. (They outgrow sensitivities but not allergies.) If you or the baby's father or your other children have food allergies or sensitivities, or are prone to eczema, then your baby is more likely to be food sensitive, too. Symptoms of a food sensitivity include cramping and abdominal pain, bloating, foul-smelling gas, diarrhea, eczema, incessant fussiness, vomiting, and constant congestion or colds.

Even if you have a Naugahyde palate, think of your baby's

palate as velvet. She may easily be sensitive to foods you eat without a second thought.

If your baby is sensitive to a food in your diet, it affects his ability to nurse. Muscles respond to allergic reactions, and since the tongue is a muscle, an allergic baby may have a hard time using his tongue to suckle.

Signs of food-sensitivity reactions include fussiness, skin rashes, red cheeks, diarrhea, vomiting, and congestion. If you've eaten something that provokes a sensitive reaction in your baby, she'll probably react within 3 to 6 hours after your meal. If your baby is sensitive to citrus, it may take 1 to 4 hours for the citrus allergen to show up in your milk and only a day for that allergen to build to a level she finds intolerable. She may react while she's still nursing or up to 4 hours later. Certain allergen-provoking foods remain in your system and enter your milk several days after you've eaten them.

The dietary culprits that provoke sensitive reactions include milk and dairy products, soy, eggs, peanuts, wheat, fish, corn, and citrus. It's not unusual for a baby to be sensitive to a food you craved and ate throughout your pregnancy, like tomato sauce. Babies also can be sensitive, but not allergic, to other foods: Broccoli, onions, cabbage, carbonated soft drinks, and caffeinated sodas or coffee can make a sensitive baby gassy.

You can reduce the risk of food sensitivities by breastfeeding exclusively until your baby is 6 months old and then introducing solids carefully, and by avoiding allergenic foods in your own diet if you see food-sensitivity symptoms in your baby. Learn to read labels closely. Like foods that contain casein, lactose, and other dairy derivatives, many food products contain extracts from eggs, fish, peanuts, and soy.

To ferret out an offending food, keep a diary of everything you eat and drink, including seasonings, or follow an elimination diet: Start by avoiding a particular food (e.g., cow's milk and all foods made with milk or milk solids) for 10 days to 2 weeks. If the baby shows no change by then, try eliminating other foods, one at a time. Some babies may react to garlic, curry, and other spices, so try to eat only three or four single-ingredient foods at a meal. (Instead of a Thai curry, choose the grilled chicken and rice noodles; order rice and beans instead of a fajita with all the fixings.) Within a few days, you'll be able to see the relationship between the foods you eat and your baby's reaction.

Usually, only one or two foods are the culprits. You don't need to follow a drastic elimination diet. Instead, cut out the most likely suspects, such as dairy, wheat, and peanuts. Because certain allergen-provoking foods remain in your system and can enter your milk several days after you've consumed them, you must strictly follow elimination diets for at least 10 days. If the baby's symptoms clear up within 10 days, try reintroducing the eliminated foods, one at a time and 1 week at a time. (If you eliminated dairy and wheat, start eating cheese OR bread again—not a cheese sandwich—until you've been able to monitor the baby's reaction for a week.)

If you have to eliminate a whole food group, like dairy, ask your doctor for advice on nutritional supplements or alternative foods; it may help to consult a registered dietitian as well.

See also Allergies, Dairy; Allergies and Sensitivities, Soy; Foods to Avoid

Sample Food Log

	Time of Snack	Breastfeeding Session	Reaction	Urine/Stool
Midnight-1 A.M.				
1 A.M. to 2 A.M.	1:30 — 8 oz. skim milk	1:15 to 1:40	fussy	wet diaper
2 A.M. to 3 A.M.		2: 10 wakes w/rash		
3 A.M. to 4 A.M.				
4 A.M. to 5 A.M.		4:30 to 5		4:40 runny stool
5 A.M. to 6 A.M.				
6 A.M. to 7 A.M.				wet diaper
7 A.M. to 8 A.M.	7:30 - grits, pat butter			
8 A.M. to 9 A.M.		8 to 8:40	fussy; still has rash	
9 A.M. to 10 A.M.		9:15 to 9:25 (comfort?)		
10 A.M. to 11 A.M.	10:30 - skim milk shake			
11 A.M. to noon		11:20 to 11:45	very fussy, gassy	11:30 runny stool

Allergies (Yours), About

Some nursing moms with allergies find relief by closing the windows, cranking up the air conditioning, and rubbing a topical menthol ointment, like Vick's Vapo-Rub, on the temples and sinus area. (If you use an ointment, wash your hands thoroughly afterward.) The ointment seems to work as a temporary remedy, calming down allergic reactions so a mom can concentrate on nursing instead of blowing her nose.

SPECIFIC MEDICATIONS

Allegra: No data are available on its transfer to breast milk. A similar product, Seldane, is also based on fexofenadine, and studies on Seldane indicate that only a minimal amount is transferred to breast milk.

Claritin: About 0.02 percent of what the mother ingests is transferred to her milk, according to the limited research available. Claritin is used for children, so it is considered safe for breastfeeding mothers.

Nasal sprays: Most nasal sprays are safe for nursing moms. Some nasal spray contents have been linked to impaired linear growth of the fetus, so don't use them if you are pregnant while nursing.

Seldane: *See* Allegra

Allergies, Dairy

Q: My 3-week-old daughter has diarrhea that, according to my pediatrician, is the symptom of an allergic reaction to milk products I've eaten. I've eliminated milk from my diet as well as my prenatal vitamins. But she's still having diarrhea. What am I doing wrong?

A: Diarrhea in a breastfed baby looks and smells different from a normal mustard-colored stool. Twelve or more poopy diapers within 24 hours, with watery foul-smelling stools, indicate diarrhea and require seeing a pediatrician immediately.

Symptoms of a food allergy—more accurately called a food sensitivity in babies—include

- Constant fussiness
- Eczema (dry skin with red patches or a rash or hives)
- Diarrhea, foul-smelling gas and cramps, vomiting (especially with blood flecks)
- Bloating
- Canker sores
- Yeast infection (thrush)

A dairy sensitivity indicates an inability to digest the milk proteins in dairy products. Lactose and its various forms—milk sugar, glucose, galactose—are in many infant foods, pharmaceuticals, bakery products, sweets, and more.

So even though you've eliminated milk, it's possible that dairy products are sneaking into your diet. It may be in vitamin and herbal supplements, or a prescription drug you're taking. If that's a possibility, go to a pharmacist with a bag containing everything you're taking, over-the-counter or prescription, for help in analyzing the contents.

You must examine product labels for casein, a phosphoprotein that's one of the chief components of milk and the basis of cheese used in many food and nonfood products. A list of other culprits:

- Milk solids ("curds")
- Whey
- Sodium caseinate (the most common form of caseinate) or any other ingredient that includes caseinate
- Sodium lactylate
- Lactalbumin (and anything else that begins with "lact")
- "Nondairy" (a phrase that indicates less than 0.5 percent milk by weight and does NOT mean milk free)

And be cautious of generalizations like "natural ingredients" (a catchall that can include dairy products and by-products), "hydrolyzed vegetable protein" (casein may be used in processing).

Are you keeping a food diary? Different symptoms can mean

different food allergies, and babies who are allergic to one food can be sensitive or allergic to another. A baby who is dairy sensitive may also develop soy allergies, especially if exposed very early to soy in a formula. Go back to your pediatrician and discuss the problem with her.

If your baby is sensitive to dairy products, he may outgrow it by the time he's 5 or 6 months old, especially if you're cautious about your diet. By 6 months, an infant's bowel has matured enough to digest and absorb complex food and is less at risk for food sensitivities.

See also Allergies (Baby's), About; Colic; Lactation Consultant; Latching On, About; Thrush, About

Allergy Medications and Breast Milk

Q: I'm breastfeeding my 6-week-old, and I suffer from intolerable seasonal allergies. When I was pregnant, I took triamcinolone acetonide (sold as Nasacort). But the product literature cautions nursing moms who want to use triamcinolone acetonide. Another nasal spray, Flonase, poses the same problem. My doctor suggested Chlor-Trimeton, but it makes me so sleepy that I can't drive or concentrate well. Is there anything I can take?

A: Nasal steroids, like the brands you mention, are the safest and most effective preparations to relieve allergic symptoms in nursing mothers. Nasal sprays are considered topical therapy, and the amount your system absorbs is fairly low.

In order for a drug, or anything else you ingest, to enter milk, it must attain significant plasma levels. Nasal steroids rarely reach detectable levels in plasma. Generally, nasal sprays are safe for breastfeeding mothers. (Even oral and intravenous steroids are OK if they're used briefly and in low doses.)

The package literature you mention is published primarily as a first defense against litigation; it rarely provides accurate information for nursing mothers.

See also Allergies (Yours), About

Allergies and Sensitivities, Soy

Q: Our 1-year-old daughter can't tolerate cow's milk, and when I was nursing, I had to cut out most dairy products from my diet, too. We're weaning her from breast milk to soy milk, but she even seems sensitive to that—very gassy, with lots of hiccups, and she drools excessively. (She could be teething, though.) Could she be sensitive to both dairy and soy?

A: Yes. More babies are sensitive to dairy than to soy, but soy products are a close second to dairy products in terms of babies' allergies. Study the product labels to make sure that any solid foods don't contain soy. This can be tricky. Obviously, soy is in soy sauce, soybeans, and soy oil, but did you know it's also in some cheese substitutes and in many Asian and vegetarian food products? Soy also may be listed as tofu, edamame, soya, vegetable protein, or textured vegetable protein. Since your daughter has so many sensitivities, why are you weaning her? No formula or other substitutes, including rice milk, can provide the benefits of human milk. If you continue nursing her, you'll need to be careful about your own soy intake, since she's demonstrated a sensitivity to soy products. Ask your pediatrician to refer you to a registered dietitian, who can advise you on what foods to eat and what to avoid. The American Dietetic Association has a booklet, *Food Sensitivity,* which includes recipes along with a list of ingredients to avoid.

And take heart: Most babies eventually outgrow food sensitivities.

Almond Milk

Q: I've heard that sometimes almond milk can be an alternative for formula. Is that true?

A: Almond milk is NOT an acceptable alternative for human milk or formula. It is inadequate nutritionally, and it can be dangerous. Giving your baby almond milk now may leave her prone to a nut allergy later. Most pediatricians advise against giving a baby nuts or nut products until age 2. Human milk is best for babies and children who can't tolerate formula. If you can't breastfeed, ask your pediatrician about donor milk from a human milk bank. Donor milk requires a prescription. If that's not an option, and you cannot breastfeed, research the formula brands to see which best suits your baby.

See also Formula, About; Milk Banks, Receiving Milk from

American Academy of Pediatrics Guidelines

Q: At my son's 9-month checkup, I told the pediatrician that I planned to continue nursing for at least a year. He was surprised, and told me that most babies aren't breastfed that long. He also told me that babies get the most benefits from breast milk during the first 6 months. Should I keep nursing? I thought doctors recommended nursing for at least a year.

A: The American Academy of Pediatrics (AAP) recently extended its recommended length of nursing time from 9 months to 1 year, and advises that babies start solid foods by 6 months of age. The World Health Organization supports breastfeeding even longer than that.

Technically, your doctor's right: Most women stop breastfeeding within the first couple of months, usually because they have logistical problems. If you're happily nursing, keep it up! Breast milk continues to provide immunities and other benefits, no matter how old your baby is.

In 1997, the AAP's journal, *Pediatrics,* announced its new policy: The AAP "recommends breast milk as the preferred source of feeding for almost all babies for at least the first year of life." No matter how old your baby is, each time he nurses he will receive benefits, including antibodies. Studies by the AAP have found that breastfed babies are less are colicky, better nourished, are more resistant to infections and illnesses, and thrive better than formula-fed babies.

Antibacterial Nursing Pillows

Q: I've been researching nursing pillows, and a friend suggested buying one that's recommended as antibacterial. The brand has "bacteria-inhibiting fiberfill," and the manufacturer says it's the only nursing pillow that protects babies from germs. Is this just a marketing line, or does it really work? It'd be worth the extra money if it really does prevent infections.

A: The antibacterial line is a marketing gimmick. According to infectious disease epidemiologists at the Centers for Disease Control, antibacterial items such as sponges, children's toys, soap, and nursing pillows can't combat viruses, which cause most illnesses. You're better off buying a generic washable nursing pillow and throwing it in the washing machine a couple of times a week.

Antibodies in Breast Milk

Q: What exactly are the antibodies in breast milk? Is the foremilk more important, or the hindmilk?

A: About 80 percent of the cells in breast milk are macrophages: cells that kill bacteria, fungi, and viruses. Human milk has scores of ingredients—scientists still haven't identified some of them—not found in formula.

One reason why breastfed babies have fewer illnesses than formula-fed infants is that human milk transfers the mother's antibodies to disease to the baby. Breastfed babies are more resistant to dozens of illnesses, including ear infections, pneumonia, botulism, bronchitis, staphylococcal infections, influenza, German measles, lymphomas, and Crohn's disease. Your body produces antibodies specific to diseases present in their environment, so your milk is custom-made to fight the cold your husband brings home from work or your older child's runny nose.

Foremilk is high in sugar and low in fat. It's thin, and it's designed to keep your baby well hydrated. It is crucial for your baby to have the hindmilk as well as the foremilk because the hindmilk is rich in nutrients and fats essential to growth and brain development. Your baby needs both.

The fatty hindmilk also contains mucins, which aren't antibodies but do help the body fight off infections. A breastfed baby's digestive tract contains large amounts of *Lactobacillus bifidus,* a beneficial bacteria. Newborns have "leaky" guts, with little or no mucosal lining. The mucins in hindmilk help keep their guts lined, preventing viruses from entering. Mucins are part of a complex defense system of muscular fighters: In laboratory tests that isolated mucins from breast milk, the mucins alone killed rotavirus, one of the most common causes of diarrhea in infants.

Antidepressants and Breastfeeding

Q: I've heard that St. John's wort is the herbal equivalent of Prozac, which I took for a year before my pregnancy to treat depression. I know I can't take Prozac and continue nursing. What about St. John's wort?

A: Neither Prozac, a prescription antidepressant, nor St. John's wort, an herbal over-the-counter supplement, is recommended for breastfeeding mothers.

As yet, no research indicates that St. John's wort is compatible—or incompatible—with breastfeeding. However, without knowing how much may leach into breast milk, it's better to avoid St. John's wort. Remember, "herbal" doesn't mean "safe." Some preparations of St. John's wort are in the family of an inhibitor that has serious side effects, including seizures, photosensitivity, gastrointestinal irritations, fatigue, and restlessness.

Better antidepressant options are Zoloft and Paxil, both prescription drugs that are safe for nursing mothers to take. Zoloft is safer, according to Thomas Hale's *Medications and Mother's Milk,* but both drugs leach only negligible amounts into breast milk.

Antihistamines

Q: Before I was pregnant, I used to take Benadryl when hay fever made me miserable. Now, 2 months after my daughter's birth, my sinuses are acting up again. But the nurse told me that Benadryl could dry up my milk. Is this true? The last thing I need is to reduce my milk supply!

A: Benadryl will not always dry up your milk, but it does have that effect on some moms. Any time you take an antihistamine, you should drink extra fluids. Dimetapp is recommended to breastfeeding moms because it's less drying than Benadryl. Try to avoid giving more than two doses per day, or for more than 48 hours. Avoid the longer-acting antihistamines, which tend to be more drying than the short-term (4-hour) type.

Signs of decreasing milk supply: fussiness at the breast, increased nursing, decreased wet diapers. If the wet diapers start to look yellow, or if there are urine crystals, stop the antihistamines at once, and boost your fluids.

See also Allergies (Yours), About

Arching Baby

Q: My 5-week-old son is extremely sensitive. He tends to be very tense and alert. He arches his back a lot, especially when he's nursing and even on the changing table. He nurses all the time, but he is still gassy and burps a lot afterward, wailing and arching his back. How can I get him to calm down and nurse?

A: Arching is not unusual, but it certainly can wreak havoc with a breastfeeding relationship. Some babies can be so tight and tense that only their head and bottom, or head and heels, touch the surface they're lying on. This is not typical, and can be indicative of high muscle tone or other conditions that should be explored with your son's pediatrician. These babies tend to be exquisitely sensitive to light and noise and are easily distracted when they nurse.

There are many reasons why babies arch. Some are easily overstimulated by noise, lights, and activity around them. They need a calm, quiet atmosphere for nursing: dim lights, no music or TV, any siblings in another room. Try swaddling the baby, and avoid talking when he's concentrating on eating. Arching and the symptoms described here are also common when a baby has gastroesophageal reflux. Talk with your pediatrician to rule that out, or to treat it.

A baby who arches must be calmed before he can nurse. He probably would like to be swaddled—with his feet uncovered—because swaddling helps anxious babies feel more secure. Swaddling a tense baby is tricky: Ask your lactation consultant to show you how to swaddle your baby, and have her supervise you until swaddling is easy for you, too. Lightly wiping his face with a damp cool washcloth or a damp warm washcloth may help calm him, too. When you hold him to nurse, make sure his feet don't touch anything. If you have trouble getting him to latch on, put gentle pressure on his chin with the pad of your thumb or index finger, but stop if he resists. Forcing him to open his mouth will only strengthen his resolve to keep his mouth clamped shut.

The football position is best for a tense baby because it holds him snugly against your body. (*See* Positions, About.) Ask your lactation consultant to show you other positions that swaddled babies like. If the arching persists, ask your pediatrician if it's possible that your baby's skull and spine bones may be slightly misaligned. During birth, a baby's soft, flexible bones can slip and compress nerves, causing problems ranging from sucking difficulties to hypersensitivity. The situation can resolve itself as the baby grows, but it may take 3 or 4 months. If this is the case with your baby, ask about cranial-sacral physical therapy to realign the bones.

Sometimes arching is an allergic reaction to something in your diet. You can try an elimination diet and see if his behavior changes when you drop dairy products or other foods that tend to upset a baby's tender digestive system. (*See* Allergies [Baby's], About.)

If your baby arches only while nursing, it may be related to an overactive letdown. Does your son gulp and choke when he nurses? (*See* Overactive Letdown.)

And buy yourself some peace and time by investing in a baby swing. Hypersensitive babies usually love baby swings because the combination of position and motion has a calming effect.
See also Colic; Gas, Burping; Positions, About; Reflux

Armpits, Swollen

Q: My milk came in 2 weeks ago, and the flesh around my armpit is swollen and painful. It makes breastfeeding difficult. Is this normal? How can I reduce the swelling without losing my milk supply?

A: Actually, the tissue in your armpit area is part of the breast—it's called the tail of Spence. Your milk ducts extend from just below your breast to your armpit, so when your milk comes in, that tissue often is engorged, too. Try packing some raw, crushed green cabbage leaves between your shirt and your swollen armpit area to relieve the swelling. Once you're past engorgement, the swelling goes down and the problem should go away.

But if you still have discomfort or difficulty nursing because your armpit area seems to have extra tissue, your problem may be an inadequately fitted nursing bra. A bad bra sets you up for endless frustration, including mastitis and plugged ducts. Ask your lactation consultant to recommend a good bra-fitter.
See also Breast Lump; Cabbage Leaves and Engorged Breasts; Engorged Breasts; Mastitis, About; Nursing Bras, About; Plugged Ducts, About

Aspirin

Q: I get migraine headaches. If I take aspirin, will it affect my 7-month-old baby?

A: Aspirin is transferred to breast milk in very low concentrations, peaking about 3 hours after you take it. The American Academy of Pediatrics recommends that nursing moms use aspirin sparingly. Other pain relievers are more compatible with nursing, including ibuprofen and some prescription medications. Ask your doctor about the latter if ibuprofen is ineffective.

Asthma Medications

Q: I'm slightly asthmatic, and I use an albuterol inhaler that my doctor says is OK for a nursing mother. When the asthma gets bad, I use Pulmicort. Is that safe to take while I'm breastfeeding?

A: Pulmicort (budesonide) is powerful but reaches only a minimal level in plasma. That's true of other inhaled steroids. Their transfer to your breast milk is minimal.

Beta-2 drugs, such as albuterol, also have negligible plasma levels and are not, as your doctor noted, contraindicated for nursing mothers.

Baby Carriers, About

Baby carriers are a real godsend. Whether you use a sling, a front carrier (like a Snugli) or a back carrier (like a baby backpack or cloth wrap) depends on your baby's age, what you're doing, and what works best for you.

SLINGS

Lots of nursing moms love slings. Slings are so ample that they virtually swaddle a baby, with enough material left over to camouflage any maternal skin exposed when you're nursing. (Because it's so versatile—it's a carrier, a baby hammock, a cover-up!—a sling is the most breastfeeding-friendly baby carrier.) Once you're comfortable wearing the baby in a sling, you can use both hands for other tasks. And slings, unlike most other carriers, are so supportive that you can use them with a newborn.

Downside: Newborns and older babies may dislike the sling

because they feel lost in all that cloth. (A new mom may dislike her sling for the same reason.) It takes a while to get the hang (so to speak) of wearing a sling. At first, you'll worry that the baby might fall out, and instinctively support her with your hands, defeating the sling's purpose. If you want confidence, ask a mom who relies on a sling to help you through the beginning. Call a local branch of the La Leche League, or ask for help from someone who rents breast pumps.

FRONT CARRIERS

For newborns, you'll want the kind that has a papoose-board–type padded back and a small seat, or a seat with adjustable snaps. (Larger carriers are meant for babies who've developed neck control.) Front carriers keep babies close and snug. Convertible front carriers allow you to wear the baby facing toward your chest, or facing out—a nice alternative when the baby is older and interested in the world beyond your shoulders.

Downside: Front carriers can be awkward for large-breasted moms. Some front carriers aren't supportive enough to carry newborns. It takes time to get the knack of fastening all those straps—a new mom may find herself so tangled that she feels like Houdini on an off day. And even with a front carrier meant to be nursing-friendly, actually shifting into nursing position involves minor acrobatics. Get used to slipping a burp rag between yourself and the baby to cut down on the amount of cumulative spit-up on the front carrier. They also get awfully warm in hot weather.

BACK CARRIERS

There are two kinds of back carriers: backpacks and those modeled after the fabric swaths used in many cultures. African women, for example use an enormous length of cloth that cradles the baby in the middle, with the ends snaking under the woman's arms and tied across the top of her breasts. The Baby Wrap is the best-known brand of the African model. Its inventor, an African woman who worked as a nanny, modified the concept to include a sewn-in seat and Velcro tabs on the tie ends. African-style wraps are comfortable, and even though your baby is on your back, she rides so high that you can make eye contact by turning your head.

Downside: African-style wraps are unfamiliar to many women in the United States. A lactation consultant, a member of a local La Leche League group, or a staffer at a maternity specialty shop may be able to show you how to wear a Baby Wrap or how to tie a length of cloth to imitate the original version. (If that fails, you may have more luck by going to a business run by Africans, like an Ethiopian restaurant or an imported African artifacts gallery, for help.) Another disadvantage of wraps: You can't nurse while wearing the baby, although the wrap is a good cover-up while you're breastfeeding.

BACKPACKS

Baby backpacks are cute, and fathers love them, especially dads who feel silly wearing a Snugli or a sling, or pushing a stroller. But most baby backpacks lack head and neck support, and many manufacturers caution against using them until your baby can hold up his head (usually, about 4 months old). Look for backpacks that have shoulder straps as well as a waist belt, to keep the baby secure.

Downside: No eye contact. Nursing with the backpack on is impossible. You must be diligent about battening down all the hatches, especially the shoulder straps, because babies can fall out if you trip or lean forward. Another disadvantage: A backpack offers your baby unparalleled access to your hair. It's hard to pry off that little death grip, which can be incentive enough for a crewcut.

See also Slings and Breastfeeding

Baby-Friendly Hospital Initiative

Q: What is the Baby-Friendly Hospital Initiative? Does it mean that I won't have to worry about nurses sneaking formula or glucose to my baby?

A: The Baby-Friendly Hospital Initiative (BFHI) is a breastfeeding-friendly project jointly sponsored by UNICEF and the World Health Organization. Its goal is to encourage increasing breastfeeding rates and setting a global standard for maternity services.

The UNICEF/WHO BFHI was launched in 1995, and has been adopted by hospitals in Australia, Brazil, China, the Philippines, Scandinavia, British Columbia, and elsewhere. In the United States, hospitals have been slow to adopt the BFHI. If the hospital you've chosen has not participated in the BFHI, ask these questions to see whether its policies parallel the initiative's principles:

- Is there a written breastfeeding policy, which is routinely communicated to all health staffers?
- Are all health care staffers trained in the skills necessary to implement that policy?
- Are all pregnant women informed of the benefits and management of breastfeeding?
- Do staffers help mothers begin breastfeeding within 30 minutes of birth?
- Are mothers shown how to breastfeed and how to maintain lactation even during separation from infants?
- Is there a rooming-in policy, allowing mothers and babies to remain together 24 hours a day?
- Does the health care staff encourage breastfeeding on demand?
- Does the health care staff avoid giving pacifiers (dummies, soothers) to breastfeeding babies?
- Does the hospital encourage breastfeeding support groups and recommend them to mothers upon discharge from the hospital?

The Baby-Friendly Hospital Initiative also suggests a list of questions for physicians:

- Does the waiting room include materials or images that present breastfeeding as a natural way of feeding babies?
- Do the physician, the staff, and other patients feel comfortable when mothers nurse in the waiting room?
- Does the physician inform all pregnant women of the benefits and management of breastfeeding?
- Is the physician aware of breastfeeding support groups in the community? Does the physician provide references to them?
- Does the physician feel competent in supporting mothers as they establish and maintain lactation?
- Can the physician address breastfeeding problems? If not, can the physician refer a nursing mother to an expert who can?
- Does the physician rarely recommend complementary feeding or weaning as a management strategy?

For more information about the Baby-Friendly Hospital Initiative, visit http://www.aboutus.com/a100/bfusa/index.htm

Babywise

See Ezzo, Gary; Schedules for Feeding and Infant Management Programs, About; Scheduled Feedings

Bactrim and Breast Milk

Q: My doctor prescribed Bactrim for me. Is it safe for me to take Bactrim, or will it leach into my breast milk?

A: Bactrim, a combination of Trimethoprim and sulfamethoxazole, is excreted into breast milk in low concentrations. For healthy, full-term infants and older nursing babies and toddlers, those concentrations are considered safe by the American Academy of Pediatrics. However, sulfa drugs can cause problems for preemies and for babies with glucose-6-phosphate dehydrogenase deficiency or hyperbilirubinemia. The medication's levels peak in the milk 2 to 3 hours after ingestion, so try to schedule your doses and nursing sessions around those peaks.

For additional resources concerning prescription and over-the-counter medications, see the Appendix.

Bathing Suits

Q: I will be nursing my daughter over the summer, and I want to buy a bathing suit that's breastfeeding-friendly. Are there special suits for nursing moms?

A: Swimsuits, unlike bras, rarely need much modification to be breastfeeding-friendly. Usually, you can free one breast just by lifting it out of the cup. Arrange a lightweight baby blanket over one shoulder for discretion—it will be less stifling than a towel.

If you really want a swimsuit designed for breastfeeding, some companies make them. They're available at maternity stores and through companies that sell nursing bras.

See also Nursing Bras, About; Appendix

Benadryl

Q: About 3 days ago, when I had a bad cold, I took Benadryl. Afterward, I noticed a reduction in my milk production. I think it was caused by the Benadryl. Is there an alternative antihistamine that won't affect my milk supply?

A: Antihistamines in general, including Benadryl, may decrease your production of milk. But if you take antihistamines for only a few days, it shouldn't affect your milk supply much longer than that. Breastfeeding mothers should avoid antihistamines for the first 6 to 8 weeks of nursing, or use the drugs for as short a time as possible.

To counter the antihistamines' effect on your milk supply, nurse frequently—at least every 90 minutes. If your nursing sessions are spaced more than 3 or 4 hours apart, express your milk, either manually or with a pump. Drink plenty of water—10 8-ounce glasses of water a day—to counter the antihistamines' dehydrating effect.

After you've stopped the antihistamines, your milk supply should rebound within 72 hours.

See also Allergies (Yours), About; Medications and Breast Milk

Birth Control, About

Most forms of birth control will not affect your milk supply.

Two exceptions: Conventional birth control pills and all intrauterine devices (IUDs) except for copper IUDs. The hormones in conventional birth control pills leach into your breast milk, and the estrogen can lower your milk supply. In fact, Stilbestrol, a synthetic estrogen, was once used in injections to "dry up" milk, but its use was discontinued because of its connection to endometrial cancer and other cancers. Most IUDs release hormones that are incompatible with breastfeeding.

Breastfeeding-friendly birth control includes

- Lactational amenorrhea. If your periods haven't resumed, if you're nursing exclusively and frequently (if you are not supplementing or going more than 4 hours between daytime feeds and 6 hours between nighttime feeds; and your baby is younger than 6 months old) then breastfeeding can be a form of birth control. Problem: if just one of those conditions changes, you can easily get pregnant. Studies have found that a breastfeeding woman is more likely to have an anovulatory menstruation (a menstrual period not preceded by ovulation) when her cycles resume.
- Copper IUD. The copper interrupts your normal reproductive cycle by causing the lining of your uterus to shed frequently, but it leaves your milk unaffected. Problem: Slightly increased risk of uterine infection and rupture.
- Depo-provera, a progesterone formula injected every 3 months. Problem: Once you've received the injection, it is effective for at least 3 months. Lactation consultants advise nursing moms to try the mini-pill before using

Depo-provera. There are other contraindications. Ask your obstetrician about them.

- Mini-pill, a progesterone-only birth control pill. Problem: The mini-pill is compatible with breastfeeding, but it does have other side effects. Again, ask your obstetrician about it.

Birth Control by Breastfeeding

Q: I'd prefer to avoid giving my 4-month-old a sibling for a year or two. I don't want to use condoms, and I know I can't go back on the pill. Is it true that you can depend on breastfeeding as a form of birth control? For how long?

A: Breastfeeding is not a substitute for birth control, even when your baby is breastfed exclusively—no bottles, no solids. If your breast milk is your baby's sole source of nutrition, your body responds by going into lactational amenorrhea: your menstrual periods cease. But it's not foolproof. Ideally, if you're nursing full time (at least once every 6 hours), breastfeeding can be an effective form of birth control (98 percent). However, lactational amenorrhea depends on an exquisitely delicate balance in the breastfeeding relationship. If you're separated from your baby, even for only a few hours a day if you have a job, or if your baby uses a pacifier, it can upset that balance, and you can get pregnant. Sometimes you can ovulate, even when you're breastfeeding exclusively, and it's possible to get pregnant without resuming your menstrual periods.

Some women resume their menstrual periods even if they are breastfeeding exclusively. Once your period returns, so does your fertility, so you'll need an alternative form of birth control. Some women don't resume their periods until their baby is more than a year old, but that doesn't necessarily mean that they're not fertile. It's safest to use a second form of birth control even if you're exclusively breastfeeding.

See also Birth Control, About

Biting, About

A teething baby bites anything he can, from chew toys and frozen washcloths to your nipples. When your baby nips, it isn't malicious—but it definitely hurts. You can teach a baby to stop biting, but it takes time and patience. Some techniques:

- Say, "Don't bite Mama" in a chirpy voice to avoid upsetting the baby. (Downside: Being chirpy is tough when you're clenching your teeth.)
- For small babies (2 to 5 months): Immediately break the suction on your nipple by inserting your finger between the nipple and the baby's mouth. Take him off the breast and say, "No biting." Even very young babies (2 months or so) will catch on. It may take a week, but it's worth the effort.
- For older babies (6 months and up): Break the suction, pull away, and say firmly: "No biting. That hurts Mommy. You can eat when you don't bite me." Then give the baby a real teething object. Try nursing again a few minutes later.
- Enforce your own versions of the "three strikes and you're out" rule: If the baby bites twice, take her off the breast and say, "No biting." Wait a few minutes before letting her resume nursing. Repeat the strategy if she bites again. She'll get the idea.

You can learn to sense when she's about to bite, too. Some babies are more likely to bite during certain times of the day, especially during what one mom calls the UnHappy Hour, between 5 and 7 P.M. Pay attention when she's nursing, and take her off the breast before she has a chance to get bored.

Expect tears and frustration. The first time or two she bites, your baby won't understand why you're upset. If you immediately unlatch her as soon as she bites, she'll learn to associate biting and being taken off the breast. (She'll still cry, but out of hunger instead of confusion.)

If the baby continues biting when you try to resume nursing, put off the breastfeeding session. If the baby is old enough to eat solid foods, offer a piece of banana, some Cheerios, or easily dissolved crackers; sometimes older babies who bite while breastfeeding want to try another kind of food but don't know how to express their desire. If he's too young for solids, offer a frozen washcloth or a popsicle made from breast milk.

Biting

Q: My 5-month-old daughter has started biting when she nurses. I've tried pulling her closer, or breaking her latch with my finger (which gets her off my nipple), but she still bites when we start nursing again. How can I teach her to stop?

A: Biting does hurt. It's small consolation that this stage usually doesn't last very long.

Most babies bite only after they're sated, and sometimes they bite because they feel playful. Did your daughter accompany her nip with a big grin?

Your baby can't bite when she's fully latched on: She has to break suction first. If she's tried to bite you, watch her closely while she nurses. The instant she breaks that suction, slide your finger into her mouth. (She'll still try to bite, but she'll nip your finger instead.)

You've already tried two techniques that usually work: pulling the baby tight against you to cut off the air supply, forcing her to open her mouth to breathe; and unlatching her. You can reinforce what you're doing by telling her firmly, "No biting." She's old enough to understand.

See also Arching Baby; Biting, About; Latching On, Clamping Down; Teething

Blanched Nipples

See Nipple Blanching

Bleb

Q: I have a white dot on my nipple, on the areola, and that breast is becoming painfully tender. Is it a pimple? How do I get rid of it?

A: What you're describing sounds like a bleb: a raised dot that usually accompanies a plugged duct. If you have a plugged duct, your breast is quite sensitive, and it may be painful to nurse. More than one bleb is an indication of thrush.

See Milk Blisters; Plugged Ducts, About; Thrush, About

Bleeding from Nipples

See Nipple Pain, About; Rusty Pipe Syndrome

Blistered Nipples

Q: My 4-week-old is trying to learn how to breastfeed after being formula-fed and bottle-fed with expressed breast milk since birth. I've breastfed her exclusively for 2 days, and my nipples are covered with extremely painful blisters. She is sucking and swallowing, so the latch-on should be correct. So, why am I getting blisters?

A: It sounds as if she may not be latching on correctly. Is she taking in some or all of the areola—the pink-brown area that circles the nipple—when she latches on? Or is she only sucking on the tip of your nipple? If your nipples are blistered (sore, cut, or bright red, or look and feel like chapped lips), you probably are having problems with the latch-on or the positioning. Nipples are fraught with nerve endings. That's why they're so sensitive and so easily damaged.

She may also have a poor sucking reflex. It's easier to get milk from a bottle than from a breast, since the milk (or formula) just drips from an artificial nipple.

Have a lactation consultant watch you as you nurse. She can assess the situation and show you how to get the baby to take in more of your nipple, and teach you nursing positions that will relieve the pressure on your nipples and make it much easier to breastfeed.

See also Latching On, About; Milk Blisters; Nipple Pain, About; Nipples, Sore, About; Positions, About

Blisters, White, on Nipple

See Milk Blisters; Thrush, About

Blood, Donating

Q: Can I donate blood when I'm lactating? Or could it somehow compromise my milk supply or my health?

A: Some blood banks do not accept blood from lactating women because of the risks associated with the volume of fluid being removed. Others will accept blood from healthy lactating women, provided that their obstetricians say they're sufficiently recovered from the effects of pregnancy, labor, and delivery, and that they're drinking enough fluids to replace the lost blood. (You'll have to boost your normal fluid intake for about 24 hours during and after the blood donation.)

Blood Pressure Medications

Q: My blood pressure stayed high after birth (140/94), and my doctor put me on Accupril. Will this affect my nursing 3-month-old son or my milk supply? I noticed that for the first 3 days after I went on the medication (about 2 weeks ago), Timmy nursed constantly.

A: In "Medications and Mother's Milk," Thomas Hale writes that Accupril (quinapril) is secreted in animal milk (less than 5 percent). No documented evidence exists that the drug is secreted into human milk, but he cautions that nursing babies must be watched for hypotension (abnormally low blood pressure), sleepiness, and poor suckling.

See also Appendix

Bloody Nipple Discharge

See Rusty Pipe Syndrome

Boiling Expressed Milk

Q: Should I sanitize expressed milk by boiling it? I know that milk banks pasteurize human milk, but also I've heard you shouldn't microwave expressed milk. But is it OK to boil milk?

A: You're right: Milk banks do pasteurize donated milk with a special process called Holder pasteurization: rapidly heating the milk to 62.5 degrees Celsius, and holding at that temperature for 30 minutes. Boiling milk is not the same as pasteurizing milk. Human milk should not be boiled, and it doesn't need to be sanitized.

Milk banks pasteurize milk for health and legal reasons, since most donated milk goes to very ill or health-compromised babies. There's a significant nutrient loss when human milk or cow's milk is pasteurized. Still, even pasteurized human milk is superior to formula; vitamins A, D, and E; riboflavin; niacin; and biotin are nearly completely preserved. Vitamin C has a 65 to 90 percent survival, folic acid 60 to 69 percent, thiamin 65 to 100 percent, and vitamin B_6 88 to 105 percent. Epidermal growth factors, nonimmunoglobulin, *Lactobacillus bifidus*, growth factor, and fatty acids all are stable as well.

It is not necessary to worry about whether your own milk is sanitary as long as you take precautions to wash your hands before and after pumping, and you are diligent about keeping your pumping equipment clean.

Bottles, About

Most babies must be taught how to use bottles, just as they have to be taught to breastfeed. You may need to experiment with different nipple/bottle combinations until you hit on one that your baby likes best. Many breastfed babies find it easy to make the transition to bottles that use nipples made by Avent, Playtex, and

Evenflo. Buy only one bottle or nipple at a time until you find the kind your baby prefers. Breastfeeding advocates say that one rule of thumb in choosing bottles and nipples is to avoid products made by companies that sell formula, reasoning that the elongated, less natural nipples make it so much easier for a baby to drink that she'll be disinclined to work for the milk from real (or realistic) nipples. (There's more than a grain of truth to that logic, though it's also true that unflinching breastfeeding advocates would rather breastfeed a newly teething baby than give their money to formula companies.)

The alternative: nipples and bottles from companies that produce, sell, and rent breast pumps.

When to introduce a bottle depends on your circumstances. If you're planning to be a stay-at-home or work-at-home mom, you'll need breaks. A caregiver will have an easier time if your baby accepts a bottle. Most lactation consultants advise against offering a bottle until a baby is at least 6 weeks old. But some moms wait until the baby is 4 or 6 months old and then find that the baby pushes away the bottle. If a baby is initially reluctant to accept a bottle, slip the rubber nipple between her lips after she's fallen asleep while nursing. It can help her get used to the new texture. Teaching a baby to take a bottle can require persistence and patience.

Try experimenting with the milk's temperature. Some babies will accept milk or formula only if it's body temperature; others prefer it cool or even cold.

It's a good idea to introduce a bottle before it's absolutely necessary. If you're returning to work outside the home, experiment with bottles 2 or 3 weeks before your first day back. Do not offer the bottle yourself. Another caregiver—your spouse or a babysitter—should offer it; a breastfed baby nearly always prefers milk directly from her mother. Babies have a keen sense of smell, and you'll probably have to leave the house during the bottle experiments.

Infants can be susceptible to nipple confusion—a term that's something of a misnomer. Babies with nipple confusion aren't confused: They prefer artificial nipples to the real McCoy.

Breastfed babies also sometimes have trouble with bottles because the pattern of sucking is different. Breastfeeding requires a baby to open her mouth wide, and her tongue to move past the lips as the baby performs a lip-suck movement, while efficient bottlefeeding requires a closed-mouth position with the tongue remaining inside the mouth. Babies use a combination of suction and compression for both breast- and bottlefeeding. If your baby has this problem, try using a sippy cup.

See also Nipple Confusion; Overfeeding

Bottles and Nipple Confusion

Q: I have a 2-month-old baby, and I'll be returning to a part-time job soon. I want to leave my husband, who'll be caring for our son, some bottles of expressed breast milk, but I'm worried about nipple confusion. Are some commercial nipples more realistic than others?

A: Nipple confusion is less likely for a 2-month-old than for a 2-day-old. Arrange for your husband to handle a few feedings before your first day back at work, so he and the baby can establish their own routine and iron out the first few bugs.

Many moms like Avent bottles and nipples. Evenflo's and Nuk's orthodontic nipples and angled nursers also get high marks in breastfeeding focus groups.

One mom cited an advantage of the Evenflo orthodonic nipple: It has a large base that requires the baby to put more in his mouth, so the baby doesn't have to chew on the nipple to get milk. She liked that because the transfer from bottle to breast was smooth and because they avoided nipple confusion (and its consequences, which include sore, cracked, and bruised nipples).

See also Nipple Confusion

Bottle, Introducing

Q: How long should I wait before giving my newborn a bottle? I worry about nipple confusion, but I don't want her to reject a bottle when she's 4 months old and I'm returning to work. And I also worry that if she takes a bottle, she won't want to nurse any more. Is that possible?

A: Since your baby is a newborn, wait until she's 6 weeks old before introducing a bottle. That will reduce the odds of nipple confusion. If you nurse her for 4 months, she's likely to continue nursing even if she gets supplementary bottles during the day. Try having your spouse or another caregiver offer a bottle—when you're out of the house—once or twice a week. That will help her get used to bottles without threatening your nursing relationship.

Bottle, Refusing

Q: I just started working again, and my 3-month-old won't take a bottle from her caregiver. She cried and went without any food for 6 hours. I'm at my wit's end. Quitting my job isn't an option. Any suggestions on getting her to take a bottle?

A: How exasperating for you and your caregiver—and how tragic for your baby! Many breastfed babies initially balk at accepting a bottle, especially when other aspects of their daily routine change. As she gets used to the new schedule she may be more willing to take a bottle. Until then, here are some tips:

- Wait until the baby is actively hungry—rooting around but not crying—before offering a bottle.
- Make sure the milk is at body temperature. Heat it in a bowl of hot water, not on the stove, and never in the microwave oven.
- Try holding the baby in different positions. Some babies prefer to be cradled as if they're nursing, but other babies accept bottles only if they're facing away from the caregiver or sitting in a bouncy seat—something

very different from their customary breastfeeding position.

- If the baby repeatedly turns away from the bottle, don't force it. Try again later. Forcing the bottle into her mouth will teach her to hate and fear bottles and to reject them even more vehemently.
- Try giving her expressed milk with a medicine dropper, spoon, or sippy cup.
- If your baby is gaining weight appropriately and producing the requisite number of wet and poopy diapers each day—8 to 12 for babies a week old or older—but still refuses to take a bottle in your absence, it's possible that she's among the babies who'd rather skip eating until they can be breastfed. This makes for busy nights and evenings for you, with marathon nursing sessions. You'll need help. Ask for it, and accept it.

See also Bottles, About; Diaper Count

Bowel Movements

See Stools

Bras, Nursing

See Nursing Bras, About

Breast Compression

Q: My newborn either falls asleep at the breast or has trouble latching on. My nipples are sore, and she's not gaining well. What can I do to encourage her to latch on and stay that way?

A: Breast compression is one way to continue the flow of milk to the baby when the baby is not actively suckling. It simulates, and stimulates, a letdown reflex by causing your milk to flow. Breast compression is especially helpful for babies who fall asleep while nursing, who have poor weight gain, who have colicky behavior, or who feed frequently and/or at length. It also helps mothers with sore nipples and those with a history of blocked ducts or mastitis.

To compress your breast, hold the baby in one arm and your breast with the other hand. Put your thumb on one side of your breast and your fingers on the other side, well back from the aureola. Latch on the baby, and wait until she begins suckling.

When she stops actively suckling—you won't feel that open-pause-close suck—compress your breast by squeezing gently. Don't squeeze so hard that it hurts, and try to avoid changing the shape of your areola. After a squeeze or two, the baby should start suckling again. Continue the pressure on your breast until the baby stops suckling. When she stops suckling, she may start again once you release that pressure. If she doesn't start nursing again, repeat the compression.

Continue until the baby stops nursing even when you compress your breast. Allow her to stay latched on a bit longer in case she decides to nurse on her own. Otherwise, let her come off the breast, or unlatch her. If she's still interested in nursing, you can repeat the process with your other breast.

See also Latching On, About

Breast Implants

Q: I had breast-enhancement surgery, with saline-filled breast implants, a few years ago. Now I'm expecting my first child. Can I nurse her?

A: Your success at breastfeeding will depend on the techniques your surgeon used. Incisions placed under the breast fold or near the armpit are least likely to damage the milk ducts and nerves. Incisions closer to the areola—like the half-moon cuts on its outside edge, with the implants slipped behind the chest wall muscle tissue—can make breastfeeding more problematic. Studies have found that incisions made close to the areola can sever the milk ducts and nerves.

Have a lactation consultant work with you and evaluate your milk supply and production in the first few days after your baby's birth as you're establishing breastfeeding. If you are able to breastfeed, keep a close watch on your baby's intake and output. Count how many wet and poopy diapers she produces in 24 hours, and monitor that, along with her weight gain, in a notebook. If she's gaining appropriately and producing 8 to 12 wet or poopy diapers, you'll be fine. Otherwise, you may need to supplement.

See also Diaper Count; Lactation Consultant

Breast Infections, Duration of

Q: First, I had a blister on my left breast. Then I got a plugged duct, and then mastitis. Even though I continued nursing and massaging the lump until it was gone—and I'm still on antibiotics—that breast is still tender and painful. How long should this go on?

A: You should feel the effect of an antibiotic within 24 to 72 hours. It's possible that the antibiotic your doctor prescribed isn't doing the job. It is also possible that your infection is complicated by something else. See your doctor again, right away, and ask her to reevaluate your condition.

See also Abcess, Breast; Mastitis, About

Breast Infections, Preventing

Q: When my daughter was 4 months old, I came down with mastitis. No warning: I just woke up with a fever and chills and a breast that felt as if a mule had kicked it. The antibiotics worked like a charm. But I came down with mastitis and two plugged ducts before she weaned. I don't want to go through this with the baby I'm expecting next month. How can I avoid more infections?

A: Prevention is definitely the best cure for mastitis and other breast infections. Technically, garden-variety mastitis is not an infection—it's an inflammation. The milk proteins distending the alveoli and surrounding blood vessels and tissue prompt your immune system to react as it would to a foreign protein—by fighting back. Your pulse rate goes up, your temperature rises, and you feel lousy.

The last thing you'll want to do is nurse, because the affected breast hurts too much. But the best cure is to nurse as an old-time Chicago voter was purportedly advised—early and often. If you don't nurse on the inflamed breast, you're probably going to end up with infective mastitis, and ultimately a breast abscess.

Most breast inflammations and infections begin with positioning problems. Even a baby a month old or older, one who's already got the hang of breastfeeding, sometimes doesn't nurse properly, especially if the mother produces so much milk that the baby hardly needs to suckle. If he doesn't have to work to get the milk, the baby may not suckle well enough to squeeze all the milk out of the sacs. (One scenario: The remaining milk builds up, stretching the milk-secreting cells and other tissue, and you wind up with plugged ducts, a breast infection, or mastitis.)

A tender red patch on your breast is the first warning sign of inflammation. To prevent inflammation and infection, get the blocked milk flowing. Put warm, damp towels on the tender breast. Massage the blockage by using the pads of your fingers to stroke the area from just above the tender spot to the nipple. Stroke the affected area, gently moving your fingers toward the tip of your nipple, as the baby is nursing and between nursing sessions. It will hurt—but a breast abscess hurts more, and the only cure for an abscess is surgery.

See also Abscess, Breast; Mastitis, About; Plugged Ducts, About

Breast Lump

Q: After nursing my daughter for 3 months, I noticed a lump just below one nipple. I'm reluctant to allow a biopsy because the lump is so close to the nipple that I'm afraid it will affect my milk ducts. Is there another way to check whether it's cancerous?

A: Lactating breasts tend to be lumpy, but the situation you describe shouldn't be put on hold. It is not necessary to wean your baby in order to diagnose the lump. A fine-needle aspiration can be done without compromising your ability to breastfeed, and there are other diagnostic procedures that won't interfere with your milk production.

Odds are that the lump you've found is a galactocele, a milk-filled cyst. Your breast tissue and milk ducts extend to your armpit—it's called the tail of Spence—and it's not uncommon for part or all of that area to become engorged. An ultrasound procedure can determine the location and content of the lump.

It's a good idea to nurse your baby just before undergoing a breast exam, or any other diagnostic exam, to reduce the amount of milk in your breast. Then you'll be more relaxed, and it will be easier to perform the diagnosis.

Other breast changes that require prompt evaluation:

- Lump or thickened area in your breast or underarm
- Change in the color or texture (wrinkle, puckering, scales) in the skin of your breast, nipple, or areola
- An unusual discharge from your nipple
- Change in the size or shape of your breast

See also Prefers One Breast; Lopsided Nursing; Rusty Pipe Syndrome

Breast Shells, and Leaking

Q: I'm wearing breast shells to un-invert my nipples. The problem is that the shells make my breasts leak incessantly. Even wearing nursing pads, I have to change my bra and top every 2 or 3 hours! Is this supposed to happen?

A: No, it's not. There are two kinds of breast shells, also known as milk cups. They look almost identical, so read the small print on the packaging, if you've got it. Yours should read "For inverted nipples." The other kind reads "For sore nipples." Make sure you get the right kind.

Breast shells are plastic and dome-shaped, with a central opening. They have an inner ring that goes around your nipple;

the dome goes over that. When the shell is positioned over an inverted or flat nipple, it exerts a suction that draws the nipple through the center hole. (Sort of like pasties, only not sexy.)

The shells for flat or inverted nipples are designed to press on the areola—the pink or tan skin around the nipple—and stretch the fibrous tissue that makes your nipple flat. Pressing against the areola will make your breasts leak, because the shell also exerts pressure against the milk sinuses just behind the areola. The shells for sore nipples are meant to keep your bra and clothes from rubbing against sore nipples. If you've got the right kind of breast shells, examine them closely. If the shell has a spout-shaped hole in the exterior, arrange it so that the spout points up instead of down. That will minimize the leaking.

Breast Shells vs. Nipple Shields

Q: I'm pregnant with our second child, and I want to breastfeed. I also tried to breastfeed my son when he was born, 2 years ago, but couldn't because I had flat or inverted nipples. Someone suggested breast shells or nipple shields. Which kind should I get? Where do you find them?

A: Breast shells—as opposed to breast (or nipple) shields—are a two-part saucer dimpled with holes. One part goes directly on your breast, pushing your nipple through a large opening. The dome-shaped top acts as a protective layer, preventing fabric from putting pressure on your nipples. Breast shells work by gently pressing the areola , encouraging the nipple to protrude.

If you know you have inverted nipples, you can start wearing breast shells in your second trimester (unless you previously have had a miscarriage; the shells exert enough pressure to stimulate contractions). After your baby is born, you can wear breast shells between feedings. You can't wear breast shells while you nurse, so be watchful when the baby latches on to make sure that he opens wide and gets a mouthful of nipple and areola. Caveat: Breast shells don't always work. Ask a lactation consultant or nurse-midwife to suggest other interventions.

Nipple shields are a different beast altogether. They're silicone nipples that cover your own nipples and are meant to be worn as you nurse. The problem with nipple shields is that they can cause nipple confusion, just as bottles do, and babies can become so dependent on them that they refuse to nurse without a nipple shield. In extreme cases, nipple shields can save a breastfeeding relationship. Caveat: Weaning a baby from nipple shields is sometimes a long process.

See also Breast Compression; Nipples, Inverted; Latching On, About; Nipple Shields; Nipples, Sore, About; Positions, About

Breasts, Differing in Size

Q: After I nursed my first child, my breasts became lopsided. The right one is more than two cup sizes larger than the left. Even after weaning, my breasts didn't return to proportion. Now, nursing my second child, the difference is bigger than ever. The large breast leaks constantly, and the small one makes less milk. How did this happen?

A: It's not unusual for breasts to be different sizes, and if one breast produces more than the other, the baby tends to prefer to nurse on that side—which only exaggerates the size difference. Usually, the breasts return to size.

In many cases, when breasts are asymmetrical, there is a connection with the drug diethylstilbestrol (DES), a synthetic estrogen that was given to 5 to 10 million pregnant women between 1938 and 1971. Daughters of women who took DES often have asymmetrical breasts (shaped differently and sized differently) as well as other health problems. One solution: Wear a falsie, and consider plastic surgery after you're certain you don't want any more children.

Breasts, Large, and Latching On

Q: My breast is bigger than my baby's head. (I'm a 38DD.) It's impossible to get her to latch on correctly, with all of the areola in her mouth. How do other large-breasted moms cope with nursing?

A: One trick you can try during the early days of breastfeeding is to roll up a receiving blanket and put it under your breast, to help lift it. Another trick is to fix a fabric sling for your breast: Use an Ace bandage or a scarf, and tie it around your neck. This makes it a lot easier to bring a large breast up to the baby's level. It also helps to make a sandwich out of your nipple: Fold your areola around your nipple, and get as much as possible into her mouth. (It's okay if not all of the areola fits into her mouth.)

See also Latching On, About

Breasts, Returning to Size

Q: After I wean my baby, will my breasts return to their prepregnancy size? My husband loves the fact that I'm so well endowed, but I hate it. On the other hand, I'd rather look like this than have a couple of big empty bags hanging on my chest.

A: Breast size changes with age. Changes in size and shape—sagging or flattening, increasing or decreasing in bulk—are due more to genetics than to breastfeeding.

Most women find that pregnancy causes visible changes in breast size and that their breasts grow again when lactation is at its peak. As you taper off breastfeeding, your breasts will decrease in size again, though not necessarily to their prepregnancy size. Some women stay large, and others go from a D cup to an A cup. Your breasts normally will maintain some fullness, at least until menopause.

Breast Size, Large

Q: Even before I was pregnant, I had very large breasts—38D. Now, in my third trimester, I'm 38DDD, and I know it's only going to get worse. It seems that moms with normal-sized breasts have the easiest time breastfeeding. I look at some of the pictures of nursing moms in my baby books, and they're all much smaller than I am. My right breast already is the size of a full-term baby! Should I just pump, instead of trying to nurse?

A: The size of your breasts doesn't have any effect on their ability to produce milk. Small breasts and large breasts all have the same number of glands and milk ducts. The size is related to fatty tissue. If it's any comfort, there are moms who wear J cups and are nursing 11-month-old babies!

The good and bad news: Size-wise, it'll get worse before it gets better. Your breasts will feel like watermelons when your milk comes in, and it'll take a while before your breasts and your baby establish their equilibrium. But this lasts only a few days to a couple of weeks. Then your breasts will stop feeling so hard, and if you continue nursing for more than a couple of months, your breast size will decrease too. Have faith in your body.

Breasts, Sagging After Nursing?

Q: My sister says that breastfeeding will stretch your breasts and leave them saggy after the baby weans. I'd still nurse my baby even if I thought I was going to look like a tribal elder in an old *National Geographic* photo, although I don't much like that prospect. Is she right?

A: Congratulations on establishing a successful nursing relationship. You're right: Breastfeeding does not cause breasts to sag or stretch. (Time does.) Your breasts will change, but pregnancy affects them more than breastfeeding.

Breastfeeding in Public, About

Many new mothers, and some experienced moms, have a hard time breastfeeding in public. Because you're self-conscious about what you're doing, especially if you've had trouble getting your baby to latch on, or if you have a baby who's easily distracted, you may feel as if everyone in the vicinity is watching you.

The truth is, few people are even aware of what you're doing.

If they do notice a mom holding a baby, they'll assume she's resting or comforting the baby, and go on with their business.

It's easy to understand why women are reluctant to nurse in public. In a culture that views breasts as erotic and is also hypersensitive about any connection between children and sex, a mother who nurses her baby in public is especially vulnerable to tension and embarrassment.

Breastfeeding in public is protected by law in about half the states in the United States. Even in states and municipalities that lack such laws, nursing mothers are rarely disturbed. (If a passerby, business owner, or manager asks you not to breastfeed, chances are that you'll be left alone if you stand your ground instead of slinking away.)

It helps to act confident. A woman unbuttoning a shirt is more likely to be noticed than a woman who seems to be adjusting her top. Practice latching on the baby quickly, easily, and nonchalantly. Practice at home in front of a mirror, or have your spouse or a girlfriend watch to reassure you of your discretion.

If you feel uncomfortable unbuttoning a shirt or lifting a top, consider buying one of the nursing tops sold in maternity stores and at children's consignment shops. They're expensive, but worth the investment if they make you feel more comfortable.

Tip: You can also make your own version of nursing tops by using two oversized T-shirts. In one, cut two breast-level openings. Wear that shirt under a second T-shirt, and just pull up the outer T-shirt when you need to nurse.

Another trick: Pin together two receiving blankets along one edge, with a gap large enough for your head. When it's time to nurse, pull the blankets over your head. One blanket will cover your front, and the other covers your back. Both drape along your side, so you and your baby are covered from all angles. Even babies who don't like to nurse with a blanket overhead will tolerate this arrangement if they're really hungry.

The only way to be comfortable breastfeeding in public is to go ahead and do it. The most secluded places for breastfeeding in public are department store dressing rooms. Look in the infant and toddler's section, where many stores have baby rooms. Lots of malls have a toddlers' play area, with comfortable benches or chairs that are perfect for nursing. And if your baby is going through a growth spurt, nursing almost constantly, go to the movies. Movie theaters are ideal—they're dark, and everyone is paying attention to what's on the screen, not what's happening among the audience.

See also Nursing Tops

Breastfeeding in Public, Being Discreet

Q: I try to nurse my 8-month-old son at home because I feel so self-conscious breastfeeding in public. Sometimes it's unavoidable. I try to be discreet, but I still feel as if people are staring. Any tips on how to avoid onlookers?

A: Try to focus on what you're doing, without being furtive. Remember, most people around you are preoccupied with their own business. If they notice a woman sitting with a baby, they'll first assume she's resting. Find a quiet bench or chair, and settle the baby in nursing position. Then get him latched on. Oversized shirts or nursing shirts provide the best coverage.

If you use a sling, that's a nearly foolproof way to camouflage a nursing baby. Even large babies can seem a bit lost in all that yardage, and the sling can be positioned to cover up whatever you bare.

See also Breastfeeding in Public, About; Nursing Tops

Breastfeeding in Public, and Husband's Disapproval

Q: I don't mind breastfeeding in public—I'm pretty discreet, and the only time anyone could see my breast is during the latch-on—but my husband doesn't want me to nurse where everyone can see me. How can I convince him that it's not the same as a peep show?

A: Personal modesty is something instilled in each of us during childhood, and some people are much more modest than others. In your husband's case, his modesty extends to his feelings about your body as well as about his own. It may not be possible to change the way he thinks and feels.

However, perhaps you can offer some solutions that he'll find agreeable. You can try nursing in your car instead of outside at the park. At the mall, borrow a dressing room (maternity stores are especially sympathetic to nursing moms). At a restaurant, sit in a corner booth with your back to the other diners. And who knows? Eventually your husband may realize what you already have discovered: Breastfeeding a baby isn't the same as flashing your boobs. Once you've gotten your baby latched on, most people won't even give you a second glance.

See also Breastfeeding in Public, About

Brewer's Yeast

Q: Is it safe to take brewer's yeast to increase my milk supply? A friend told me she increased her milk supply dramatically by taking 3 tablets 3 times a day.

A: Brewer's yeast has no harmful effect on breast milk, but no medical studies verify its reputation as a galactagogue (substance that promotes the flow of milk). Brewer's yeast, like fenugreek and other popular milk-enhancers, works for some women and not for others.

See also Milk: Low Supply?

Bubble Palate

See Palate, High

Burping a Sleepy Baby

Q: My 4-month-old daughter wakes in the morning with lots of gas. When she sleeps in our bed, she wakes my husband and me with a reveille of "two-bun salutes." I think she wouldn't be so gassy if I could get her to burp after our late-night nursing sessions, but she usually falls asleep. How can I get her to burp when she's asleep?

A: It's tough, but possible, to burp a sleeping baby. Try sitting her on your lap, with your hand cupped under her chin to support her head and chest. Pat or rub her back for 4 or 5 minutes. If she needs to burp, she can burp even if she's asleep. If she hasn't burped after 5 minutes, she probably won't burp at all.

Could she be gassy because of a foremilk/hindmilk imbalance at night? Does she nurse long enough at night to get to your hindmilk, or does she tend—as many babies do—to fall asleep at the breast? If that's the case, her gassiness is because she's getting too much foremilk.

See also Foremilk and Hindmilk

C

C-Hold

Q: I have large breasts, and I heard that the C-hold is best for supporting my breasts. Which hand do you use?

A: The C-hold uses your outside hand (the hand on the same side you're nursing) to support your breast. Place your palm gently under your breast, with the edge of your hand as close to your chest as possible. You may need to hold it slightly away from your chest in order to support your breast adequately. Form the letter C with your hand. Be careful to keep your fingers away from the areola—fingers that are too close may interfere with the baby's latch. He won't get enough areola in his mouth to get at the milk sinuses behind the areola, and your nipples will be sore. Support your breast lightly—think of your hand as a pillow, not a C-clamp. If your grip is too hard, it can damage your breast tissue or cause a clogged duct.

See also Positions, About

Cabbage Leaves and Engorged Breasts

Q: My breasts are so engorged and tight that they're like watermelons. I heard that cabbage leaves will relieve the pain. What kind of cabbage? Raw or cooked?

A: Engorgement can be painful when you're weaning. (If you're not weaning, your breasts may be engorged because your baby isn't emptying your breasts when she nurses; have a lactation consultant observe a nursing session if your breasts are always engorged.) Raw cabbage leaves can help relieve painful, swollen breasts. In terms of effectiveness, it doesn't matter whether you use green or red cabbage, but for practical reasons, use green cabbage; red cabbage can stain your clothing.

To make a bra salad, crush the cabbage leaves with a rolling pin to make them pliant enough to mold against your skin. Plaster a layer of leaves completely over each breast—you will feel a little like a jolly green giantess—and keep the leaves in place with a stretchy exercise bra or a towel tied sarong-style. Rest with the leaves in place until the leaves wilt. Keep a washcloth or towel handy if you start to leak heavily. Do this twice a day, not more. This ought to relieve the engorgement pain by the second or third day. If the pain persists, see your doctor.

Some women get large lumps in their armpits 2 or 3 days after childbirth. Cabbage leaves will help that, too.

There's an old wives' tale that cabbage leaves can dry up your milk within a day or so, because many moms use cabbage to relieve breasts swollen from weaning, but no medical research supports this. Still, some nursing mothers report that prolonged or routine use of cabbage leaves can diminish their milk supply. Use cabbage leaves sparingly, not on a regular basis.

See also Weaning, About

Caffeine, Effect on Breast Milk

Q: I've avoided caffeine in coffee and cola ever since I became pregnant, and then after I started nursing. Sometimes I have a decaffeinated coffee when I go out. I'd like to have a real coffee once a day, two or three times a week, but will this harm my baby?

A: That's the $64,000 question for any nursing mother who longs for caffeine to propel her through sleep-deprived days.

Caffeine is approved by the American Academy of Pediatrics for breastfeeding mothers. Only a small amount is secreted into breast milk. The average cup of coffee contains 100 to 150 milligrams of caffeine, and peak levels of caffeine are found in breast milk about an hour after you've had the coffee. The average dose of caffeine your baby gets is less than 3 milligrams per kilogram daily, if you're a moderate coffee drinker (5 cups or less of coffee or other caffeine-containing beverages, painkillers, stimulants, etc., per day).

Caffeine has a half-life of 80 hours in a newborn, a bit less in babies up to 3 months old, and 2.6 hours in babies 6 months old. It can cause irritability and insomnia, so watch your baby's reaction to a full-strength cup of coffee before you embrace old habits.

Calcium in Mother's Diet

Q: Do I need to boost my calcium intake when I'm breastfeeding? I've heard I should be eating lots of cheese, yogurt, and whole milk or 2 percent milk. Normally, I eat maybe 8 ounces of yogurt every other day or so, and during pregnancy I drank about 12 ounces of milk a day. Is that enough?

A: That much milk will provide you with enough calcium. (Nursing mothers need 1,000 to 1,200 milligrams of calcium daily.) But you don't need to drink milk in order to make milk. Remember that many babies are sensitive to milk and other dairy products. In most of the world, nursing mothers drink no milk at all but rely on soy, fish, greens, and grains for calcium.

Calcium Supplements for Babies

Q: I heard that cow's milk has much more calcium than human milk. Should I give my baby calcium supplements?

A: An ounce of human milk contains about a fourth as much calcium as an ounce of cow's milk. That may be why babies fed with dairy-based formula tend to grow larger and heavier during the first year of life than do breastfed babies. However, formula-fed babies also excrete a lot of unused calcium. Breastfed babies retain more of the calcium they take in. A healthy breastfed baby does not need calcium supplements.

Calories, Estimating Daily Requirement for Nursing Mom

See Weight Loss

Candy, Effect on Breast Milk

Q: I know I should eat more nutritious food, but the truth is I eat candy when I'm hungry, and I don't have time to cook. My 6-month-old daughter is already plump, and I'm worried that she might inherit my tendency to gain weight. Is it possible that all that sugar is increasing the calorie content of my breast milk?

A: All nursing moms tend to have the same proportions of protein, fat, and carbohydrate in their milk, with lactose (milk sugar) being the chief carbohydrate. There is little evidence to show that a sugary diet affects the nutritional composition of breast milk. The calorie count for an ounce of breast milk ranges from 18 to 25.

In other words, your sugary diet is not causing your daughter's plumpness. Breastfed babies often tend to be plump during the first 6 months and then stretch out into slim toddlers. Research indicates that breastfed babies may be less likely to become obese during childhood.

You already know this, but your eating habits aren't doing you much good. Candy is nutritionally empty. You're setting yourself up for a sugar slump that will hit almost as soon as you've finished your snack. Try replacing your snacks with air-popped popcorn, grapes, a banana, rice or popcorn cakes, nuts and raisins, or a bagel. It's just as easy to fix a nutritious snack that will satisfy your appetite for something crunchy or sweet.

Casein

Q: My baby is sensitive to dairy products, so I've cut everything with casein out of my diet. Then I learned that human milk contains casein too. Why does she tolerate the casein in my milk but not in cow's milk?

A: Human milk does contain casein. Breast milk is low in caseins A, B, and C relative to the caseins in cow's milk. And not all digestive systems are equal: Yours may digest casein efficiently, while your baby has trouble with the additional casein that cow's milk adds to one casein or another in your milk.

See also Cow's Milk; Allergies, Dairy; Allergies and Sensitivities, Soy

Cesarean Section and Breastfeeding

Q: My baby will be born by cesarean section, and I'd like to nurse right away. I'm worried about the pain from the incision. How can I hold the baby in a way that won't hurt (too much)?

A: Here are a couple of tricks from other c-section veterans. If you want to try holding the baby across your lap, put a pillow over your knees and part of your stomach. That will help keep pressure off the incision. If you're nursing in bed and feel as if you're straining, prop several pillows behind your back so you're lying on an incline.

The football hold is a little different from the cradle hold but much easier on the incision. Sit on a couch or bed, or a wide chair with low arms, with a pillow pushed up against your thigh. Lay the baby on the pillow, with the baby's chest against your side and the baby's head facing your breast, and latch her on.

See also Positions, About

Cesarean Incision and Delayed Milk

Q: My son was born by c-section 2 days ago, and my milk still hasn't come in. Another mom who gave birth (vaginally) the same day was pumping milk 24 hours later! Will I be able to nurse?

A: Yes. Be patient. Sometimes it takes a bit longer—3 to 5 days—for your milk to come in. Be patient, and persevere: The colostrum you have now is perfect for your son.

See Colostrum

Chicken Pox Vaccine

Q: I am still nursing our 12-month-old son. I'd hoped to wean him naturally, but I want to become pregnant, and when my obstetrician learned I've never had chicken pox, he recommended that I be vaccinated before trying to get pregnant again. Will I have to wean my son before getting the shot?

A: Your obstetrician probably was concerned that you may expose your unborn baby to chicken pox early in pregnancy, and likely suggested that you have the chicken pox (varicella) vaccine before you become pregnant. When a pregnant woman is infected with chicken pox, the fetus also develops the disease (congenital chicken pox), which can result in birth defects: abnormal limbs, or eye and skin defects. Exposure to chicken pox before the 20th week of pregnancy results in birth defects in 2 to 3 percent of the population. However, if a pregnant woman is exposed to chicken pox during the last week of pregnancy, it puts the unborn baby's central nervous system at risk.

The varicella vaccine (Varivax) is 70 to 90 percent effective in preventing chicken pox. Have your blood tested before getting the vaccine to be sure you're not already immune to chicken pox. (About 80 percent of adults who think they've never been exposed to chicken pox are immune to it.)

Because it is a live strain, the varicella vaccine is unlikely to transfer to breast milk. However, if you or your doctor is concerned about the vaccine affecting your 1-year-old, consider vaccinating your son at the same time.

Children's Books and Breastfeeding Images

Q: I am looking for some children's books that show babies nursing, so I can prepare our toddler for her baby sister. Can you suggest any titles?

A: Sure: *Breasts* by Genichiro Yagyu (Kane/Miller Books) is a forthright book about breasts and breastfeeding meant for toddlers and young children. The La Leche League International catalog (847-519-7730) lists more than 80 books that feature human mothers (and some animal mothers) nursing their babies. Among them: Susan Winter's *A Baby Just Like Me* (DK), *Feeding Babies* by Chiyoko Nakatani (Puffin Books), *I Love My Mommy Because* by Laurel Porter-Gaylord (Dutton Children's Books), *My Mama Needs Me* by Mildred Pitts Walter (Lothrop, Lee and Shepard), *One Round Moon and a Star for Me* by Ingrid Mennen (Orchard Books), *The Same but Different* by Tessa Dahl (Viking Kestrel), and *Over The Green Hills* by Rachel Isadora (Greenwillow Books).

Cholesterol

Q: I knew your cholesterol levels are higher when you're pregnant, but it's 2 months since my baby's birth, and my cholesterol's still borderline high. Usually I'm pretty fit. Should I be worried?

A: Not unless your cholesterol level reading is higher than 240 milligrams per deciliter. According to a 1985 study reported in *Obstetrics and Gynecology,* lactating mothers have a mean cholesterol level of 207. A reading between 200 and 239 is considered borderline high.

However, even though the desirable cholesterol level reading is under 200, the study found that lactating mothers usually have an increase in "good" cholesterol: HDL, which helps protect against clogged arteries and related diseases. After you wean, your cholesterol should return to its prepregnancy level. Still, if your total cholesterol levels are very high, or if you have a family history of artery and coronary disease, ask your doctor about having a thorough workup that measures your HDL and LDL levels and the ratio of HDL to LDL. You may need to adjust your diet as well.

See also Appendix

Cigarettes

See Smoking and Breastfeeding.

Cleft Lip and Breastfeeding

Q: My newborn has a cleft lip. The pediatrician says that we'll have to wait until she's at least 3 months old before it can be corrected. Will she be able to breastfeed?

A: Yes, she probably will. Unlike babies with cleft palate, a baby with a cleft lip—a separation of the two sides of the lip, and often the upper jaw bones or gums—actually can latch on more easily than a baby with a normal lip. Because the cleft can accommodate more of the nipple and breast tissue, she'll be able to establish good suction.

Still, you should seek help from a lactation consultant who's experienced in working with cleft lip and cleft palate babies. She can suggest the best nursing positions for your baby's particular cleft, and make sure that the latch-on is secure and strong.

Cleft Palate and Breastfeeding

Q: My 2-day-old son was born with a cleft palate. I was hoping to breastfeed, but he has a hard time latching on. If he does latch, a lot of the milk comes out his nose. The pediatrician's sympathetic, but she's told me most babies with cleft palates end up on formula. Is there any chance I can nurse him?

A: It's enormously challenging to breastfeed a baby with a cleft palate, the fourth most common birth defect in the United States. A cleft palate is an opening in the roof of the mouth, caused by failure of the two sides of the palate to fuse as the baby was developing in utero.

The wider the palate, the more difficult it is for the baby to latch on, and for you to position the nipple so the milk goes down his throat and not up into the palate opening.

A baby with cleft palate may have other issues as well. The cleft affects the soft palate's muscles, which are crucial for suckling, swallowing, and chewing. Only surgery can repair the cleft, and most pediatric surgeons prefer to wait until a baby is at least 8 months old before operating.

Still, it's possible to breastfeed a baby with a cleft palate. An aid called a palatal obturator is enormously helpful; ask your pediatrician about it. You will need to work with a lactation consultant experienced in cleft palate problems. But don't blame yourself if you're unsuccessful. Breastfeeding means a lot of extra work for a tiny baby already facing an uphill battle at mealtime.

The alternative, if you're determined to give your baby breast milk, is pumping your own milk and using the expressed milk to bottlefeed the baby. Rent or buy a hospital-grade pump, and start pumping immediately to keep your milk supply ample.

A baby with cleft palate may find it easier to nurse from a bottle. You can direct the bottle's nipple farther into his mouth, and to the side of the mouth, away from the cleft. There are nipples especially designed for cleft palates. (Some babies manage with a modified orthodontic nipple that's been boiled, with an X cut into the nipple hole to help the milk to flow more freely.)

Resolving a cleft usually requires several courses of treatment, including surgery, dental and orthodontic care, and speech therapy.

For more information about cleft lip and cleft palate, and support and advocacy groups, contact the American Cleft Palate-Craniofacial Association, 1829 E. Franklin St., Suite 1022, Chapel Hill, NC 27514. The association's toll-free line is 800-242-5338, where a staffer can answer your questions and direct you to doctors and specialists in your region.

See also Pumping, About

Clogged Ducts

See Breast Infections; Mastitis, About, Plugged Ducts, About

Clumping Milk

Q: I've had mastitis several times in my right breast. I don't have it now, but the milk I pump from that breast looks almost like condensed soup. It's so thick that sometimes it can't pass through the filter in my breast pump. It looks awful. What's causing this? Should the baby be eating this milk?

A: Clumping, clotting, or coagulated milk is an indication of mastitis, so even if you're symptom free otherwise, your old nemesis is back. See your doctor as soon as possible, and bring along a sample of the clumpy milk (a laboratory analysis may be necessary).

It's safe to continue letting your baby nurse on that breast. The milk looks bad, but it won't harm your baby. As you've learned from dealing with mastitis before, nursing and pumping early and often on the affected breast is the key to eliminating a breast infection.

See also Mastitis, About; Pumping, About

Cluster Feeding and Growth Spurts

Q: My 2-week-old daughter has started cluster feeding during the day. She nurses every 30 minutes for 4 or 5 hours, and then tapers off, nursing every hour and a half to every 2 and a half hours. Is this a growth spurt?

A: If your daughter's weight gain is on target, and your milk supply is good, this could be a growth spurt. If it is, the cluster feeding will last 3 or 4 days while your milk supply adjusts to her increased demand. (If her weight gain is not up to speed, consult your pediatrician, and work with a lactation consultant, who can judge your nursing technique and milk supply.)

It may be that this is your daughter's nursing style. If it's her style, expect it to last for months. In that case, you have three choices:

1. Have a nervous breakdown. (Just kidding.)
2. Start using a sling, and get used to cooking, cleaning, and handling other functions from a crabbed, sideways position that allows your daughter to be more or less permanently latched on.
3. Ask your spouse and good friends to bring you lots of good books and movies, and plan to eat takeout for quite a while. Ignore the dishes and dust bunnies. They're not going anywhere. (And neither are you!)

Or you can order the combination platter, using something from each of those choices. Roll with it. Eventually, her nursing schedule will become less erratic, and you'll actually manage to shower and manage other accomplishments before dusk. Meanwhile, you'll be helping the local economy by keeping the neighborhood takeout restaurants in business.

See also Breast Compression; Growth Spurts, About

Cluster Feeding and Night Feedings

Q: My 4-week-old son has started nursing almost nonstop from 5:30 to nearly 11 P.M. Then he sleeps for 3 to 5 hours. Isn't that awfully long for a newborn? Should I be waking him to nurse? Is there a connection between his eating frenzies and his long naps?

A: This is a common pattern: nonstop nursing followed by a long sleep. It's a price worth paying, from the vantage of a mom who's spent many nights up with a restless newborn, especially since many babies this age have long wakeful stretches at night.

Since he's eating so steadily in the evening, you probably don't need to wake him for a nighttime or early morning feed, assuming he's gaining appropriately and producing 8 or more wet and poopy diapers daily.

A tip: When his evening nurse-a-thon is drawing to a close, introduce a bedtime ritual. You might pat his back, or sing lullabies, or stroke his hair as you rock him. He'll learn to associate the ritual with bedtime, making the transition easier on you both later on.

And a warning: Your son is on the brink of a growth spurt that may turn his nighttime routine on its ear. Sleep while you can!
See also Growth Spurts, About

Colds

See Congestion

Colic

Q: My 5-week-old daughter is almost always fussy. I burp her during and after a feeding, but she still seems distressed. Is it colic? What can I do about it?

A: Boy, that's another $64,000 question. Colic is one of a new parent's biggest worries. It's difficult to treat, because nobody knows what causes colic. The first thing to do is eliminate the possibility of a foremilk/hindmilk imbalance, which shares some colic symptoms—a fussy, gassy baby. (*See* Foremilk and Hindmilk.)

Symptoms of colic usually start during the second week of life. Babies prone to colicky behavior are relentlessly fussy, intense, extremely sensitive, and high-need. The fussiness peaks at 6 to 8 weeks of age and usually disappears when a baby is between 3 and 6 months old.

Colic is sometimes associated with a dairy sensitivity or intolerance. This type of allergy tends to run in the family. You can rule it out by changing your diet (or, if you're using formula, switching to a soy-based or lactose-free formula). If a dairy allergy is causing the irritability, your baby should start showing signs of improvement within a few days.

Some pediatricians think that an iron imbalance can aggravate colic, often because mothers continue taking prenatal vitamins and/or iron supplements after the birth. They take the vitamins or supplements because they're told to by doctors (who often haven't studied lactation), or because they figure they might as well use up the rest of their prenatals, or because they've heard that babies need the extra iron (not true in most cases).

A good lactation consultant will advise eliminating iron first, if you're taking it, because it's so much easier than going on an elimination diet. If iron is the culprit, your baby's demeanor will change within 4 days. Eliminating dairy is much more complicated: Dairy products and derivatives must be cut from your diet for up to 14 days, and you must scrupulously read labels.

If eliminating iron and dairy hasn't helped, the next step is soy and soy products—another complicated elimination diet. Soy intolerance is the second most common problem for babies, who react to a mold on the soy that (a) triggers the response and (b) is impossible to eliminate.

If you've eliminated dairy, iron, and soy, and the baby's symptoms still haven't changed, a full diagnostic workup is necessary, including your complete dietary history.

Be extremely wary if you are counseled to treat colic by switching from breast milk to formula. Breast milk is the single best food for infants. If your baby is showing symptoms of reflux (arching, crying, frequent and dramatic vomiting), talk to your primary care provider about treatment options. Recent studies suggest that colic or infant irritability may also be associated with erratic sleep/wake patterns. Babies who have a difficult time getting to sleep and staying asleep are more easily over-stimulated when they're awake, and cannot adjust to their environment. Make sure that your baby goes down for regular naps, in calm settings. The white noise of a running dryer, or even static, tuned low, from the radio, can help lull a baby—and if that fails, most babies can't resist the soporific effects of a long car drive. Then you have the problem of how to get the baby back on breast milk, building up your milk supply, and sticking to an elimination diet because your baby is even more sensitive and possibly allergic.

You need to take care of yourself as well. Make sure that you rest when the baby does. Take an afternoon nap along with your daughter, especially if she's especially colicky in the evenings and at night.

See also Allergies, Dairy; Allergies (Baby's), About; Arching Baby; Breast

Compression; Burping a Sleepy Baby; Fennel Tea; Overactive Letdown; Pulling on Nipple; Spraying Milk; Stools, Green

Colostrum, Adequate

Q: My breasts are producing only watery-looking colostrum, even though it's been 2 days since my baby was born. Sometimes she cries right after she's nursed. Is she losing weight because she's not getting enough calories from just breastfeeding?

A: Colostrum looks thin, but it's chock-full of antibodies, and it is the perfect food for newborns. Think of it as solid gold, versus gold plating. Colostrum typically lasts 3 or 4 days until your milk comes in. As long as your baby is not dehydrated (the diaper count for a baby on colostrum is one diaper per day of age: one diaper the first day, two the second day, three the third day) and has no symptoms of dehydration, just keep nursing. The mature milk will come in soon. Sometimes it takes a little longer, especially if you've had a difficult or highly medicated labor.

Most babies lose a little weight immediately after birth. As long as your daughter is back up to her birth weight by her second week of age, she's gaining appropriately.

Colostrum is clear or yellow-tinted, but so highly concentrated that your baby doesn't need much. Lactation consultants tell moms to think of colostrum in terms of drops or spoonfuls, not ounces. If she's crying, it may be for another reason. Newborns often reflexively pass stools or urine while they're nursing, so she may need a diaper change. If a baby is awake and willing to breastfeed, let her nuzzle continuously.

See also Dehydration

Colostrum, Leaking Before Birth

Q: I'm pregnant for the second time, but it might as well be the first—the whole experience has been so different. I'm 6 months along, and my breasts began leaking colostrum a couple of days ago. Not lots, but enough to leave my bra damp. With my first baby, the colostrum didn't show up until after he was born. Does this mean the baby will arrive early?

A: It's not unusual to leak a little colostrum—it will be thin and clear or yellow-tinted—especially during pregnancies subsequent to your first. This does not mean the baby will arrive early—just that the hormones are revving up. In fact, some women continue to manufacture breast milk and colostrum long after they've weaned their babies.

Colostrum vs. Glucose

Q: I'm planning on breastfeeding the baby I expect in a week, but I'm worried because I have little or no colostrum. A friend who gave birth and wanted to breastfeed had real problems when the nurses insisted on giving the baby glucose water because they said she wasn't making enough colostrum. What can I do to increase production?

A: Even if you don't notice any colostrum, your breasts are manufacturing it. Even tiny amounts of colostrum pack a powerful immunological punch. If you are concerned about nurses giving your baby bottles of glucose water or formula—a standard practice in many hospitals, and one that can wreak havoc on a nascent breastfeeding relationship—talk to your obstetrician. Tell her to provide written instructions to the hospital staff, informing nurses that you should room in with the baby (instead of sending the baby to the nursery) and specifically forbidding artificial nipples, including pacifiers and anything by bottle unless medically necessary. (For example, hypoglycemia is rare, but it endangers a baby's brain and health, and in that case, glucose supplements are important.) Written directions ("nil by mouth") from a physician are far more effective than birth plans, which may be ignored.

See also Baby-Friendly Hospital Initiative; Nipple Confusion

Congestion

Q: My baby is terribly congested, especially in the morning when he wakes up. Do you have any suggestions on how to clear his nasal passages without causing him too much discomfort?

A: Poor kid! A stuffy nose makes it hard to nurse. One answer is literally at your fingertips: breast milk. Seriously. For many moms and babies, a little breast milk works better than baby-safe saline drops, an over-the-counter alternative.

Here's how: Express about an ounce of milk into a cup or bowl. Use a syringe to squirt about half a teaspoon into each nostril, waiting a beat between squirts. Use an aspirator to snork out each nostril. Then, squirt another half teaspoon of milk into each nostril again, and leave it there. The excess will drain into his throat and won't do any harm. Breast milk can break up and resolve the congestion faster than any product on the market.

If he's consistently congested each morning, you may also want to experiment with different positions for that first morning feeding.

If you normally nurse in bed, try sitting in a glider or rocking chair, and cradling the baby in a semi-upright position (not the football hold).

It also helps to run a humidifier in the baby's room at night and to do a little detective work. If he has down pillows or blankets—which present more of a danger than a comfort to babies, who may smother in them—he may be allergic to the feathers.

See also Allergies (Baby's), About; Positions, About

Constipation

Q: My 6-week-old daughter seems constipated. I've considered using suppositories, but a friend said that something in my milk may be causing the problem.

A: How many wet and poopy diapers is she producing each day? Is she gaining weight appropriately? Or has her weight gain stalled out? If she's not gaining weight, she may not be constipated but lacking food, and if that's the case, you need to see your pediatrician or lactation consultant to diagnose the problem. A healthy breastfed baby is not constipated.

For the first 6 weeks, breastfed newborns pass a liquid stool that looks like seedy mustard, and they often produce a stool while they're nursing. After a month or so, the number of stools drops until the baby is pooping only a couple of times a day, or even once every couple of days. As a rule, newborns poop frequently (five or more stools a day), and older babies poop less frequently.

But a newborn who has fewer than four stools a day, or is producing only a stain on the diaper, is not getting enough milk. Ask your pediatrician to weigh her, and be certain to tell the doctor that you've been using suppositories.

See also Diaper Count

Contraception Methods

See Birth Control, About

Coping with Frustration, Stress

See Critics, Coping with; Discouragement, Dealing with

Cost Benefits of Breastfeeding

Q: Obviously, breastfeeding is less expensive than using formula, but now that I'm returning to work, I'm weighing the cost of pumping against introducing formula. Since I have to buy bottle paraphernalia, will it work out to be a wash, cost-wise? Or is one method actually less expensive?

A: Renting or buying a breast pump, along with bottles, nipples, etc., still is less expensive than using formula. It costs $460 to more than $800 a year to supply formula to low-income families (Tuttle and Dewey, 1996). Families who don't qualify for federal supplements spend more than twice that much annually on formula.

Breastfeeding is superior to formula in preventing childhood diseases, including cancer, diarrhea, ear infections, juvenile-onset diabetes, meningitis, and urinary tract infections. Breastfeeding reduces the incidence of premenopausal breast cancer (Lee 1997) and decreases blood pressure and stress hormone levels. For more details, e-mail lactation@juno.com and ask for a copy of "Cost Benefits of Breastfeeding" by Karen M. Zeretzke, IBCLC.

Cow's Milk

Q: At my son's 9-month checkup, the pediatrician told me to start giving him cow's milk, even though I'm still nursing and pumping. I was surprised—I thought you weren't supposed to give a baby cow's milk before 12 months of age—but she said the guidelines have changed. I'd love to give up pumping, but 9 months seems awfully early for cow's milk.

A: Conventionally, pediatricians have recommended waiting until a baby is at least a year old before offering cow's milk (whole only), to avoid triggering a dairy allergy. The curds in cow's milk can be difficult for food-sensitive babies to digest, and digestion problems can lead to internal bleeding. Does your pediatrician want your son to go on an all–cow's milk diet, or does she suggest cow's milk as an alternative to pumping milk or using formula? As long as your baby gets plenty of breast milk, a small amount of cow's milk may be OK. Ask the pediatrician to explain her recommendation.

Cow's Milk and Cooking

Q: Why does my baby get colicky when I drink cow's milk, but not when I eat pizza or lasagne?

A: Your baby may be sensitive to some dairy products. The lactose in cow's milk changes when it's cooked, as it is in yogurt, cheese, or cooked milk products like puddings or porridges. The

caseins in milk are unaltered by cooking, so babies who are truly sensitive to dairy products react negatively to cheese and yogurt as well as to milk and ice cream in their mother's diet.
See also Allergies (Baby's), About

Coxsackie Virus (Hand, Foot, and Mouth Disease)

Q: My 5-month-old daughter recently contracted hand-foot-and-mouth disease. At first, it looked like poison ivy blisters on her tongue and legs. Her tongue bothers her so much that she has trouble nursing. I'm also worried that her big brother may catch it from her. What can we do?

A: The Coxsackie virus is relatively new (discovered in the 1960s) and is common in the United States. It's highly contagious—the virus spreads through saliva and contact with the blisters on a patient's skin, and through droplets and other secretions from patients. The virus spreads rapidly in hot and dry conditions.

The symptoms include the blisters you describe—a rash that lasts 7 to 10 days—along with a fever, sore throat, headache, decreased appetite, blisters or ulcers in the throat and mouth, and a rash on the hands, feet, and diaper area. Symptoms begin to show up 3 to 5 days after exposure to the virus, and most patients recover within a week.

Because it's a virus, it doesn't respond to antibiotics. If you're nursing, you may contract the virus as well; it is highly contagious. There is no cure, but eventually it goes away.

It's likely that your son already has been exposed to the virus, but you can take these measures to protect him and others:

- Bring your child to a pediatrician immediately if he or she shows signs and symptoms of the Coxsackie virus.
- Wash your hands with soap and water each time you use the toilet, before you prepare food, after changing a diaper, and after handling stool-soiled clothing and bedding.
- Wash toys and other surfaces contaminated by the patient's saliva.

- Keep babies and children who have the symptoms of the Coxsackie virus home from day care, preschool, and kindergarten.
- Clean your house and its surroundings to discourage flies, cockroaches, and other pests.
- Parents: Bathe or shower, and change clothes after returning from work or outdoors before playing with babies and small children.

Cracked Nipples

See Nipples, Cracked

Cradle Hold

See Positions, About

Critics, Coping with

Q: I want to breastfeed my baby, who's due in a month, but my husband is the only one who thinks it's a good idea. My mother-in-law predicts I'll turn to formula before the first week is out. My sister says it's perverted to want a baby to suck my nipples. My cousin teases me (sort of) that my breasts will get so engorged I'll think they're falling off. My best friend, who had a baby last year, says nursing is so painful that she couldn't last 2 weeks. How can I get them off my back?

A: This is a tough one. Who likes criticism, especially when you're sleep-deprived, tender from labor, and learning how to be a mother?

Attitude and tone of voice make a big difference in whether your responses will be accepted or even heard. Act happy and confident, even when you feel nervous and defensive. When someone is being critical, making a joke or laughing something away can work wonders.

Practice your critic-handling remarks with another breastfeeding mom. (If you don't know one, contact the local La Leche League—it's listed in the phone book—or ask your hospital's lactation consultant if she can help put you in touch with other local nursing moms.)

Some techniques for dealing with critics:

- Deflect with the unexpected. "Oh, Auntie Mame, your hair is FABulous!" "Look at you! Have you lost weight?" "You know, that reminds me, I was about to ask what you thought about . . ." (nursery lights, snaps vs. zippers, anything but breastfeeding).
- Turn the tables. "I'm glad you care so much about the baby. I've done a lot of research; would you read (this book/article), and let me know what you think of it?"
- Cite authorities. "The American Academy of Pediatrics and the World Health Organization have done recent studies that strongly recommend breastfeeding babies, even after they're a year old."
- State the undeniable. "You feel very strongly about this." "You could be right."
- Be inscrutable. "You've given me a lot to think about." "Hmm. I'll have to think about that."

And here are two cheery answers for the most frequently asked annoying questions:

Q: "How long do you plan to nurse?"

A: "Oh, about 10 minutes or so."

Q: "Shouldn't you be doing that in private?"

A: "No, (the baby) and I need to be together to do this."

Crossover (Modified Cradle) Hold, and Large-Breasted Moms

Q: My son is nearly 6 weeks old, and I've used the crossover hold because my breasts are fairly large. My biggest problem is that I can't discreetly feed him in public, because there's no way to avoid exposing a lot of breast when I'm latching him on—no easy trick in itself.

If I'm lucky, someone will cover me while he latches, but that only calls even more attention to us! Am I stuck with this awkwardness forever?

A: The modified cradle hold works best with newborns whose moms are pretty busty, but once your baby settles a bit more—in 2 or 3 more weeks—you'll find it easier to adjust his position while he's nursing. One large-breasted mother of a 4-month-old baby still starts out with the crossover (modified cradle) hold, and then switches to the cradle hold. It takes some practice, but the result is worth the effort. And if the baby pops off, it's easier to latch her back on.

Your latch-on problems may be due to your baby's resistance to the sensation of being pushed from behind, which is how the crossover position feels from a baby's point of view. Try what works for some other well-endowed moms: Hold your baby's head by cupping the back of his neck, so your fingers extend to his ears and the bone behind the ears. (It feels a little like pressing the ears against his skull.)

It's extremely difficult to nurse unobtrusively when you're using the crossover hold. There's really no way to avoid flashing more breast. Try to sit in a private corner, with your nursing side to the wall. Wearing a loose T-shirt helps, thanks to the extra fabric, and the baby's head will block (some of) the view.

See also Positions, About

Crying After Nursing

Q: My 7-week-old daughter is breastfed on demand. Every time she comes off the breast, whether I take her off or she unlatches herself, she whimpers a little. It's not a real cry, but obviously she's not comfortable. Why is she doing this, and what should we do to help her?

A: Are you burping her immediately? Often, this not-quite-cry means a baby has gas. If you have an abundant, overactive letdown, you might try burping her a few minutes after she latches

on, against the possibility that she's swallowed some air along with the first shower of milk.
See also Overactive Letdown

Crying While Nursing

Q: Ever since he was born, my 5-week-old son has cried while he nurses—and sometimes afterward as well. This is very stressful for both of us. Is it possible that he doesn't want to nurse?

A: No: Your baby wants to breastfeed. It sounds as if he's frustrated. He may not yet understand how to breastfeed. If he's not producing the requisite number of wet and soiled diapers (*See* Diaper Count), he may not be getting enough to eat.

Is he latching on correctly? Does he latch on, take a few sucks, and pop off? He may be mad because he's not getting an immediate reward. (Babies who've been bottle-fed often have this reaction.) Try hand-expressing some milk to encourage your letdown before latching him on. If he still balks, you may want to try using a tubal feeding aid. (*See* Tube Feeding Lactation Aids.) Once he learns that suckling gets results, your own milk will flow more easily and he'll continue to nurse.

It's also possible that you have an overactive letdown, and he's crying because the milk flows too fast for him to swallow. (*See* Overactive Letdown.)

He may be crying because of gas. He may be crying because some babies just don't tolerate much. A high-needs baby is especially sensitive during the first 3 months and needs to be held a lot.

Does he cry at one breast but not at the other? During delivery, some babies are injured. It's unusual, but not unheard of, for collarbones or other bones to be cracked or broken during a difficult delivery, and a baby's bones are so soft that the injury may initially escape detection.

If he's producing lots of wet and soiled diapers, gaining weight appropriately, and hitting other developmental milestones, talk

to your pediatrician about your concerns, and rule out physical problems that might be causing his discomfort.
See also Allergy, Dairy; Colic; Appendix

Cut on Nipple

Q: I just discovered a cut at the base of my nipple. It is not bleeding, but it is an open wound. It hurts to nurse on that breast, especially because my son is teething and sometimes his tooth scrapes the wound. How can I get the cut to heal?

A: A small cut like this is painful, and it can be slow to heal. You can alleviate the pain by taking ibuprofen and by changing nursing positions. If you're not customarily using the football hold, that position is best for relieving pressure on your nipple. If nursing on that side continues to be painful, substitute a breast pump for one or more of the nursing sessions on that breast until your cut heals. (To express the most milk possible, try to pump when the baby is nursing on the other breast.)

An antibiotic cream, like Mycotracin, may help speed the sore's healing. Be sure to wipe off the cream before you nurse or pump on that side. You also can use an all-purpose nipple ointment, which doesn't need to be wiped off.
See also Positions, About; Pumping, About

Cystic Fibrosis in Nursing Baby

Q: My baby has cystic fibrosis (CF), and I wonder if it's OK to breastfeed him. I know breast milk is high in fat and that his body can't digest fat.

A: If it's diagnosed early, there's no reason a baby with CF should not get breast milk, but it requires extra effort at a time when you are frustrated and scared. Working with a lactation consultant and a pediatrician knowledgeable about CF is a must. A baby with CF, breastfed or formula-fed, needs to take pancreatic enzymes orally, in capsules. Because of the ongoing malabsorption, it may be a challenge to keep up with your son's need to nurse, especially if his weight gain and growth were low by the time he was diagnosed. Still, there are many reasons why your son should be breastfed, including protection against infection. More important for a baby with CF is the lipase in breast milk. Lipase is an enzyme that a baby with CF is unable to produce in his pancreas, so he's unable to digest fat by himself. The lipase in breast milk actually helps a baby with CF.

D

Dairy Sensitivities

Q: Even though I've cut out dairy products in my diet after my 2-month-old was diagnosed with a dairy sensitivity, he sometimes still gets those runny stools and the rash he had when I ate dairy. What am I doing wrong?

A: Odds are that he's reacting to dairy products that still sneak into your diet. Even though you've eliminated the most obvious dairy products, you could inadvertently be eating other foods that contain enough dairy products to trigger your son's sensitivity. Dairy products are used in lots of prepared foods—bread, cookies, pasta, convenience foods, and most restaurant foods—and even in "nondairy" products like Cool Whip, which contains sodium caseinate. (Some babies even react to beef in their mother's diet.)

In your case, the culprits are probably foods containing lactose, casein, and their derivatives. All milk—including human breast milk—is composed primarily of lactose and casein A, casein B, and casein C, and dairy products are responsible for more allergies and sensitivities than any single product, as you've learned. And the first signs, as with your son, include red, itchy skin (often as a rash on the cheeks and diaper area), throwing up, and stools full of mucus.

If dairy is a problem for your baby, you need to eliminate all sources of casein until he's a year old.

Start reading the nutritional contents (labeled "Nutrition Facts") on packages when you shop. Look for milk powder, casein, caseinate, whey, cheese, margarine, and other forms of dairy protein. (Some dairy-sensitive babies are also sensitive to soy; if you can, avoid soy and soy products too.) Ask for the same information about what you order at fast-food and formal restaurants. Even a small amount of dairy is enough to trigger a reaction in a sensitive baby.

Elimination diets are a hassle, but they're worth the extra trouble if your baby has a food sensitivity. Prompt reaction to your son's dairy sensitivity now could mean that he'll avoid allergies and other lifelong dietary problems later.

For the calcium you need—about 1,000 milligrams daily—turn to calcium-fortified orange juice or a calcium citrate supplement. Antacids that contain calcium carbonate, like Tums, are less easily absorbed.

See also Allergies (Baby's), About; Colic; Cow's Milk; Diet, Mother's; Stools, Green

Day Care, Estimating Milk Needs

Q: How much milk should I give my day care provider? I hate to leave too much because she just throws out what she doesn't use.

A: If your daughter is under 12 weeks old, figure that she'll want about 3 ounces of milk per feeding. If she'll be in day care from 9 A.M. to 4 P.M., start out by giving your day care provider four 3-ounce portions of expressed milk a day. (If you're worried that she may not use it all, freeze your milk in 1- or 2-ounce portions, and instruct the provider to thaw the servings one at a time.)

Be direct with your provider if you prefer that your daughter be fed on demand rather than according to a schedule, and provide written instructions for reference. Include the information about how long breast milk can be refrigerated (5 to 8 days) or frozen (up to 6 months in a refrigerator freezer).

Enlist your provider's help so you can increase or decrease the milk stock according to need. Your daughter may eat more, especially during growth spurts. She may eat less if she decides to go on a bottle strike. (You may also want to ask your provider to comfort and hold your baby, but refrain from feeding her for 90 minutes or so before your pickup time, if you want to nurse when you get home. And set up a plan for the times you're running late, so your caregiver isn't frustrated by trying to calm a hungry baby.)

See also Pumping, About

Day Care Provider Reluctant to Use Expressed Milk

Q: My day care provider flatly told me she'd rather have my 3-month-old baby on formula than breast milk. She claims there's a risk of transmitting HIV and other diseases. (I am HIV negative.) Is she right? Can she do this legally?

A: As a business owner, she has the right to set the rules about what she will and won't feed her charges. Since you're HIV negative, she has no scientific basis to fear HIV. (Even if you were HIV positive, she would be at little risk of being infected with the virus by handling breast milk.) Some day care providers prefer to use formula because it's easier than defrosting breast milk.

If you want to keep your daughter on breast milk as long as possible, you need to find a different child care provider.

See also HIV and Breast Milk

Decongestants, Compatibility with Breastfeeding

Q: I've got a bad cold. If I take a decongestant, will it leach into my breast milk? If it does, what effect would it have on my 3-month-old baby?

A: Over-the-counter drugs often consist mainly of decongestants such as phenylephrine and phenylpropanolamine, which can sometimes pass into breast milk, but rarely in significant amounts. Decongestants are used in pediatric preparations as well.

Most over-the-counter decongestants have no negative effects on your baby. Some can have the effect of drying your milk, so be sure to drink plenty of extra fluids, and take decongestants only as long as necessary.

Dehydration

Q: My 2-month-old baby doesn't want to nurse, and her urine is very yellow. She seems dehydrated, but why won't she nurse?

A: Bright yellow urine, especially if it's accompanied by salt-like deposits, is characteristic of dehydration. It is not caused by something in your milk—in fact, your milk is what she needs. But a dehydrated baby can be so listless that she lacks the energy to do what she needs most—to nurse.

Dehydration is a serious problem. It can be fatal. Infants and toddlers are so small that they can get dehydrated so quickly that you may not be aware of their condition until they get feverish and lethargic—two of the later stages of dehydration.

You can monitor your baby for dehydration by keeping track of how many wet diapers she's producing (8 to 12 in 24 hours, if you're using cloth; 6 to 8 if you're using disposable diapers). A decreased number of wet diapers, and a decreased interest in nursing or taking a bottle, can swiftly lead to dehydration. Signs of dehydration:

- Fever
- Fontanels more sunken than flat when she's lying down
- Lethargy
- Bright yellow urine, and/or crystals in the urine
- Dry, red, or sticky lips and tongue

If she won't nurse or take expressed milk from a bottle or medicine dropper, take her immediately to a pediatrician or urgent-care center to be treated.

See also Allergies (Baby's), About; Diaper Count; Hot Weather and Nursing; Water Supplements

Dental Work and Breastfeeding

Q: I need some dental work done, and I can't bear to have it done without some kind of anesthetic. Is there a safe numbing agent for a breastfeeding mom?

A: The American Academy of Pediatrics approves lidocaine as a local anesthetic for nursing mothers. Most dentists use only local anesthetics, which leave your system quickly and leach only low to negligible amounts to breast milk.

Dental X-Rays

Q: Are dental X-rays compatible with breastfeeding? My dentist says so, but he's not a lactation expert.

A: Your milk will not be affected by a dental X-ray. You can breastfeed as usual when your dental appointment is over.

See also X-Rays, Chest

Depression and Vitamin B_6

See Vitamin B_6

Depression While Nursing

Q: As soon as I start nursing my 4-week-old daughter, I have this dramatic mood swing. I feel extremely depressed, and that sadness continues for 3 or 4 minutes into the nursing session. Then it disappears. What's causing this?

A: It may be good ol' postpartum hormonal chaos. Your body is still reacting to the initial release of oxytocin as your baby begins nursing. What you describe—moodiness or sadness during the first few minutes of a nursing session—is not uncommon. It should disappear by the time your daughter is between 6 and 8 weeks old. Many new moms experience some form of postpartum depression but feel better as they become more confident about motherhood and breastfeeding.

One study, conducted by midwives, found that women who

experience temporary depression while nursing often have experienced a traumatic labor and delivery. These mood swings also can be common in women with a history of emotional, physical, and/or sexual abuse. It's a form of postpartum depression. If the depression doesn't diminish, talk to your physician about it.

Diabetes

Q: I had gestational diabetes when I was pregnant, and some of the symptoms are reappearing. Should I stop breastfeeding?

A: While you can safely breastfeed if you have diabetes, you'll need to talk with your doctor. Being diabetic means that you're more susceptible to infections, including thrush and other yeast infections. Lactating can change your insulin requirements, too.

If you were diabetic when your baby was born, you should be monitoring your baby's blood sugar levels as well as your own. (The best tests for you are Diastix and Tes-Tape, which accurately measure a lactating woman's glucose levels.)

If you are diagnosed with diabetes, talk to your doctor about how to handle your treatment. Your insulin needs are different during breastfeeding.

Diaper Bags, Breastfeeding-Friendly

Q: I'm looking for a diaper bag designed for a nursing mom—a pocket with a bottle-holder big enough for a water bottle, not a baby bottle. But all the diaper bags I've seen are made by companies that assume you're bottlefeeding a baby. Is there such a thing as a practical, non-cutesy diaper bag that has room for a mom-sized water bottle?

A: Lands End, Eagle Creek, and (online) www.weebees.com all carry diaper bags that can accommodate big water bottles (the kind cyclists and runners use) along with other baby paraphernalia. The Eagle Creek bag is constructed like a small daypack—a refreshing change from the norm.

Don't limit yourself by looking only at diaper bags. You may be happier with a small daypack or fanny pack that has a water bottle holster and enough room inside for a diaper or two, a blanket, some wipes, and a snack. One mom found the answer at a medical bookstore, where she bought a plain doctor's bag that was insulated and had handles, a shoulder strap, and lots of pockets.

Diaper Count

Q: I know babies are supposed to produce a certain number of wet and poopy diapers a day, so you know whether they're dehydrated or constipated or having diarrhea, or they're normal. So, what's the diaper count? And does it vary according to a baby's age?

A: A baby who is exclusively breastfed should produce 6 to 8 wet disposable diapers, or 8 to 12 cloth diapers in 24 hours. That's the rule of thumb as long as the baby is taking in nothing but breast milk. Urine should be clear, not yellow.

Once she starts taking solid foods or other fluids, the number changes along with her other needs.

Keeping track of wet disposable diapers can be confusing, since they're constructed to feel dry against a baby's skin. Usually, you can tell by touching the diaper. If you touch the diaper and the gel inside feels soft, heavy, or squishy, it probably needs to be changed. (A dry disposable diaper feels stiff and light.) A trick some moms use with disposable diapers: Put a bit of tissue or cloth in your baby's diaper when you change her. Check every 60 to 90 minutes to look for moisture.

Also, a newborn may produce more wet diapers, total, than a 9-month-old. Newborns in cloth diapers may need to be changed 15 times a day, compared with 6 to 8 times a day for a baby 6 weeks old or older. After 3 months, a baby's bowel movements begin changing in texture and frequency. They are more dense than liquid, and some babies produce stools only every 2 or 3 days.

Diarrhea, Baby's

Q: My 3-month-old baby has diarrhea. Should I give her formula instead of breastfeeding her? Should I give her extra liquids?

A: Infant diarrhea is a serious problem, but it occurs far less often in breastfed babies than in formula-fed babies. (Necrotizing enterocolitis, a bowel infection that often attacks premature babies, is much more common in formula-fed babies than in breastfed babies.)

If your daughter is nursing well, keep breastfeeding. Your milk contains immunities that will help shorten her illness. Nurse on demand, even if it seems as if she's nursing constantly. The American Academy of Pediatrics encourages mothers to continue breastfeeding babies who have stomach or intestinal illnesses. Breast milk is absorbed more easily than formula and is the best fluid to rehydrate your baby. Breast milk will not aggravate the diarrhea.

Ask your pediatrician before giving her supplemental liquids, such as oral rehydrating solutions.

Diarrhea, Mother's

Q: I have diarrhea, and even though I'm careful to wash my hands each time I use the toilet, I worry about infecting my baby. Is it OK to keep nursing, or could my breast milk transmit this illness?

A: By all means, keep nursing. Your breast milk is full of antibodies to the disease that your body is fighting—it's the best medicine you could give your baby. With diarrhea, as with other common illnesses (colds, sinus infections, sore throats, etc.), by the time you develop symptoms, you've already exposed the baby (and anyone else in the family) to the infection.

It's smart to wash your hands frequently and to check with your doctor if you're taking prescription or over-the-counter medications. Most over-the-counter antidiarrhea medications are compatible with breastfeeding., but some can transfer to breast milk and present problems for your baby. Drink lots of liquids

to replace what you lose to diarrhea and other symptoms. Rest as much as you can.
See Imodium

Diet, Mother's, and Effect on Baby

Q: How can I tell whether my baby is fussy because of something I've eaten, or if something else is bothering her? She's 9 weeks old, and sometimes she is fussy after I've had lunch or dinner.

A: Certain foods and drinks can enter your milk in just 20 to 30 minutes; other foods can affect babies up to 24 hours afterward.

To determine if a specific food or drink is bothering your baby, you'll need to keep a food diary of what you've eaten, with remarks about your baby's behavior. When foods in your diet are responsible for fussiness in your baby, the usual suspects are dairy, acidic vegetables and fruits (including tomatoes and tomato products, and citrus and citrus products), broccoli, cabbage, turnips, beans, onions, apricots, and prunes. If that's the case with your baby, you need to eliminate the food, and all products containing that food and its derivatives, for at least two weeks.

Fussy, colicky behavior is common in about one-third of all babies under the age of 3 months. It's possible that your baby is just fussy as she adjusts to her new world. Babies (and toddlers) seem especially cranky between late afternoon and early evening.
See also Allergies, Dairy

Diflucan

See Fluconazole; Thrush, About

Discharge, Bloody, from Nipple

Q: When I pump milk for my 4-month-old son, I've noticed that one of my breasts seems to be bleeding. Not much, just enough to tint the milk pink. My nurse-midwife ruled out thrush, but I can't figure out what this could be.

A: Bloody discharge from nipples usually is related to damaged breast tissue or to engorgement. Sometimes the milk appears to be bloody, or pink, in what's known as "rusty pipe syndrome." But rusty pipe syndrome usually clears up within a week or so, and it is more common when first-time moms are establishing breastfeeding.

The discharge may be caused by intraductal papilloma, a small benign growth on the lining of a milk duct beneath the areola.

Bleeding can also be related to pumping: Are you using a new pump? Are you routinely setting the pump at the highest level of suction? In either case, dial down the suction, and give your breast tissue a break. If there are other changes in your breast—puckering or dimpling, or scaly skin, or a change in color—you need to see a doctor.

Is the discharge spontaneous: Does it leak out on its own? Or do you notice the discharge only when you're nursing or expressing milk, or massaging your breasts? Spontaneous discharge should be evaluated immediately by your doctor. Ask her to request a laboratory diagnosis.

See also Nipples, Sore, About; Pumping, About; Rusty pipe syndrome

Discouragement, Dealing with

Q: I hate nursing! I know it's the best thing for my week-old newborn, but we're into our 7th straight day of latch-on problems, my nipples are cracked and bleeding, my breasts are like melons, and when my son does manage to nurse, I have to grit my teeth because it hurts so much. This is not the madonna-and-child experience that I'd expected.

A: Congratulations for being determined to nurse your son. Does it help to know that you've got lots of company in your misery?

Virtually all new moms have pain and problems during the first 2 or 3 weeks of breastfeeding. Usually this is because they lack help and support, or are given inaccurate advice and treatment. The first 2 postpartum weeks are difficult, not only because of the challenges associated with establishing breastfeeding but because of all the challenges a newborn presents. Some breastfeeding experts skim over this aspect of breastfeeding, concerned that moms already uncertain about their ability to breastfeed won't even give it a try.

Breast milk is absolutely the best nutrition you can provide for your son, particularly during the first 6 weeks of his development. Try choosing his 6-week anniversary as your goal for breastfeeding him. Circle the date on your calendar, and concentrate on the benefits you're providing for him when you're feeling especially disheartened.

The good news is that the first 2 weeks of breastfeeding typically are the toughest. Even moms who don't have many problems with nursing find that period a trying one. Once you make it past the halfway mark to your 6-week goal, you may find that breastfeeding is getting easier and easier.

By the time you hit the 6-week anniversary, you'll be a seasoned pro—and if, despite extensive help from lactation consultants and a pediatrician knowledgeable about breastfeeding, you're still experiencing the same level of pain and difficulty, you'll be able to switch to formula knowing that you tried your best and that your son has the benefits of a full 6 weeks' worth of antibodies. Good luck! And remember: The odds of physical, spiritual, and emotional benefits are in your favor—and your son's—if you continue to nurse, aiming at that short-term goal.

It is essential to have a lactation consultant watch you nursing, to help with your latch-on technique. If your hospital or HMO provider can't supply a lactation consultant, call the local La Leche League, whose leader can help you for free.

See also Breast Compression; Depression; Lactation Consultant; Latching On, About; Nipple Pain, About

Distracted Baby

Q: It's impossible to keep my 9-month-old daughter focused on nursing when we're away from home. She's so interested in everything that she pops on and off the breast, especially if some sound or movement catches her attention. What should I do?

A: A 9-month-old baby is full of curiosity. New sights and sounds are as interesting to her as nursing. Remember that after 9 months of breastfeeding she may be an efficient nurser—she can eat her fill in less than half the time she needed when she was 9 weeks old.

Some techniques for limiting distractions:

- Sit in a position that allows the baby to simultaneously keep an eye on the world while nursing.
- Sing or talk or make faces to keep her focused on you.
- Toss a blanket over your shoulder, and drape it over your baby's head, like a tent.
- Nurse in a quiet room with dim lights. If you're in public, look for a clothing store—dressing rooms can be ideal.
- If she still pops off, close the milk bar until she's hungry enough to pay attention.

Dizziness

Q: I get dizzy after almost every breastfeeding session. My son is about 5 weeks old, and I get so dizzy that I really worry that I might faint and drop him. Should I stop breastfeeding?

A: Some women get dizzy after nursing if they're not eating enough, or if they're drinking so little that they get lightheaded from dehydration. Are you sure that you're getting enough to eat and drink? Odds are that you're also a little disoriented from being sleep-deprived—your son is still so young that he's probably not sleeping through the night, and your body is still adjusting to being on call 24 hours a day.

Try to rest when the baby rests, and to eat small but frequent meals. And drink lots of liquids (your urine should be pale or clear, not yellow). If the dizziness still persists, see your doctor. You may be anemic or have low blood pressure.

Domperidone

Q: I'm having real problems establishing breastfeeding. My newborn has a weak suck, and my milk supply is low. Also, my nipples are sore and cracked because he clamps down so hard, trying to get milk. I heard that there's a drug that can boost your milk supply, but my doctor hesitates to prescribe it. Why?

A: Domperidone, usually prescribed to treat gastrointestinal disorders, inhibits the body's production of dopamine. By suppressing the production of dopamine, it may have the side effect of increasing the hormone prolactin, which stimulates the cells in your breasts to make milk.

The problem is that while Domperidone has boosted milk production in some women, its manufacturer does not endorse it for that purpose. The side effects are not always predictable, and individual response to drugs can vary tremendously. But this is a side effect rather than the drug's primary purpose, and few American physicians would be willing to prescribe it to a nursing mother. (Reglan [metaclopramide], which you can get in the United States, has an effect similar to that of Domperidone, but it is also unpredictable and has other side effects that seriously compromise whatever benefit it may provide.)

Some doctors do prescribe Domperidone, but only as a last resort for women desperate to breastfeed. However, Domperidone has some negative side effects, including headaches, abdominal cramps, and dry mouth. Its transfer into breast milk is negligible, so it is safe for breastfeeding mothers and babies.

There are other ways to encourage your baby to become better at breastfeeding: correcting the latch, expressing milk by hand or with a pump to improve supply, boosting your water intake,

breast compression. Some mothers swear by herbal boosters like brewer's yeast, fenugreek, and Mother's Milk tea.
See also Breast Compression; Fenugreek; Mother's Milk Tea; Nipple, Cracked; Pumping, About

Donor Milk

See Milk Banks

Doulas

Q: My mother-in-law offered to hire a doula to help me out with the baby. Can a doula help with breastfeeding problems?

A: It depends on the doula. A doula (*pronounced* dwaa-la) is a woman dedicated to nurturing and supporting new mothers and families, providing important breastfeeding support during the crucial days after birth. In traditional Greek culture, a doula was indispensable help for new parents.

The contemporary version of a doula combines traditional wisdom with practical resources and guidance. A doula may be trained in lactation issues, but she is not necessarily also a lactation consultant.

Usually, a doula works 3 to 5 hours a day for the first postpartum week or two. Expect to pay between $300 and $800 for a doula; some doulas are willing to work on a sliding scale according to your needs.

A doula instructs new parents on cord care, diapering, bathing, maternal and infant nutrition, and newborn development, and she helps mother and baby learn essential breastfeeding techniques, including latching-on tricks and different positions for nursing.

Doulas make life easier on a family with a new baby by helping with preparing meals, caring for siblings, and handling household chores. You can find out more about postpartum doulas in your area by contacting the National Association of Postpartum Care Services: 1-800-45-DOULA.
See also Lactation Consultant

Down's Syndrome and Breastfeeding

Q: My baby has Down's syndrome. Can I still breastfeed her?

A: Yes. A Down's syndrome baby benefits from breast milk, which can help improve her muscle tone and boost her immune system.

Some Down's syndrome babies nurse capably at birth. But because a baby with Down's syndrome may have poor muscle control, your baby could need extra time to learn how to latch on and coordinate sucking, swallowing, and breathing. If she is not doing well, seek out a lactation consultant experienced in special-needs babies. You can also try these exercises to encourage the suckling technique:

- Put your finger in her mouth, and gently rub her gums, stroking from the front to the back of her mouth.
- Lightly stroke downward on her throat, to encourage her to swallow.
- Trace the baby's mouth and cheeks with one finger.
- Softly pop your finger in and out of her mouth, stroking her tongue to encourage her to suck at your finger.

Learn to recognize your baby's waking signs. She'll nurse better if she's awake. You can waken her gently by rubbing the soles of her feet, changing her diaper, and patting her legs and stomach with a cool, damp washcloth.

You'll spend a lot of time feeding her. Get in the habit of stimulating your letdown reflex by expressing a little milk before putting her to the breast. Breast compression also helps with these babies. If she's reluctant to nurse, use an eyedropper to squeeze a little expressed milk into her mouth.

Experiment with nursing positions until you find one that supports her head and doesn't require her to turn to face your nipple. One position: Lay her on her side, with her arm around your waist, belly to belly with you. Then press her chin down to help her open her mouth wide as she latches on. Make sure the nipple is centered in her mouth. Her lips will be flanged—turned out in an exaggerated kiss—and if you delicately pull down her lower lip, you should be able to see her tongue between her lips and your nipple.

See also Breast Compression; Lactation Consultant; Latching On, About

Dribbling While Nursing

Q: My 8-week-old son is gaining well and nursing like a champ. My problem is that he dribbles while he nurses. Sometimes he lets milk squirt out his mouth. I have a strong letdown—milk jets out 3 or 4 feet when I express a squirt or two before nursing—that's probably related to the problem. I wonder if this is normal and if I should be concerned about the dribbling. I usually end up with a lapful of milk.

A: Sounds as if your son has figured out his own way of dealing with your strong letdown. Since he's gaining well, you don't need to worry about whether he's getting enough milk. Many moms who have an ample supply of milk notice that their babies dribble a bit when they nurse, especially when they first latch on and the letdown is strongest.

Try putting a cloth diaper under his chin to catch the overflow. That will help you avoid a damp lap. You might also express a little milk before putting your son to the breast, so the initial flow isn't quite so strong.

And an unsolicited suggestion: Since you have such an abundant supply, consider donating to the nearest human milk bank. They always need more milk, and you'd be helping babies who desperately need breast milk.

See also Foremilk and Hindmilk; Milk Banks; Leaking, About; Spraying Milk

Driving and Breastfeeding

Q: On long car trips, when there's not much traffic on the road, my sister-in-law has breastfed her babies. She's never had a problem, not even when she drove past a state trooper. Is that legal?

A: Not by any stretch. In the United States, Canada, and many other countries, it's illegal to ride with a baby in your arms instead of strapped into a car seat. (Driving and breastfeeding simultaneously is as dangerous as it is illegal.) It is possible, if you're flexible and agile, to breastfeed a baby sitting next to you in a car seat. But if you're driving, don't even try. It's worth the time and effort to pull off the road, turn off the ignition, and breastfeed the baby. Otherwise, you literally could multi-task yourself—and your baby—to death.

Droopy Nipples

See Nipples, Droopy

Drying Up

Q: How fast can your milk dry up? I still have overactive letdown, but I feel as if I don't have much milk any more. Because of the overactive letdown, I'm supposed to nurse only from one breast in a 2-hour period. However, my 6-week-old daughter can empty a breast in less than 20 minutes—it used to take her 40 to 45 minutes—and is still rooting around, acting hungry. So I break the 2-hour rule and offer the other breast, and she empties that too.

I'm feeding her constantly, but I feel as if there's nothing left for her to eat! The only time I get engorged is at night, when she sleeps for 5 hours—and then I'm torn between sleeping and pumping.

A: Don't worry about your daughter taking less time than before to empty your breasts. As babies get older they become more efficient at suckling. They can empty the same amount of milk as they did before, only in less time.

Your breasts adjust, too, to your baby's demand. The overactive letdown may have resolved itself by now. And it sounds as if your daughter also may be hitting the 5- to 6-week growth spurt. Babies tend to nurse their way through growth spurts, and that would explain her increased appetite.

It's possible that exhaustion is affecting your milk supply. Why don't you take a "nursing holiday"—go to bed for a couple of days, cuddling up with your daughter to rest and nurse as much as you can? Let the housework and other chores wait, or have someone else take care of them.

See also Growth Spurts, About; Supply Problems, About; Weaning, About

Ducts, Plugged

See Breast Infections; Plugged Ducts, About; Mastitis, About

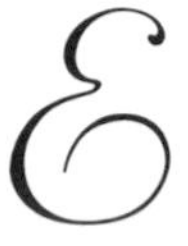

Ear Infection

Q: I've been exclusively breastfeeding my daughter, now 7 months old, all her life. I thought this would prevent ear infections, but we just got back from the pediatrician, who diagnosed her with—guess what?—a middle-ear infection. Isn't breastfeeding supposed to insure against ear infections?

A: Babies who are diagnosed with ear infections (acute otitis media) more often are formula-fed than breastfed, according to a study of 306 infants in Buffalo, New York. Between 6 and 12 months of age, 25 to 51 percent of the breastfed babies were diagnosed with first-time ear infections, compared with 54 to 76 percent of the formula-fed infants. The researchers concluded that formula-fed babies tend to be more susceptible to ear infections, and breastfed babies tend to be more resistant.

Breastfeeding your daughter, in other words, means that she's less likely, statistically, to get as many ear infections as a formula-fed baby. Exclusively breastfeeding your baby is not an iron-clad guarantee against ear infections, but it surely improves her odds against them.

Eating Enough: How Can You Tell?

Q: My 2-month-old son loves to nurse—or suckle, anyway—but I've had trouble breastfeeding him. He'll suckle for a couple of minutes, then pop off. He loves expressed milk in a bottle—he empties bottles without a problem.

So I've supplemented my nursing with expressed milk and formula until last week, when he started taking less and less of the bottle each day. Now he takes no more than 10 ounces by bottle. How do I know if he's eating enough?

A: He is eating enough if he is gaining normally, produces 6 to 8 very wet (but not yellow) disposable diapers (or 8 to 12 cloth diapers) daily, and can go a couple of hours, give or take, between feeds. He may be getting what he needs from breastfeeding alone.

Once babies figure out how to breastfeed, they can get what they need in 10 minutes or less. Taking less formula may mean that your milk production is catching up, or already has caught up, with his demand. It also sounds as if he may have had some trouble with nipple confusion. Some babies can't go back and forth easily between breast and bottle. Fluid leaks continually from an artificial nipple, while babies must suckle to elicit a steady flow of milk from the breast, so many babies find it easier to drink from a bottle. If he's not gaining well or producing enough wet diapers, nipple confusion may still be a problem. Breast compression can help resolve nipple confusion, but ask an experienced lactation consultant for help.

See also Breast Compression; Lactation Consultant; Nipple Confusion

Echinacea

Q: Is it OK to take echinacea to fight off a cold? If it leaches into breast milk, will it help my baby stay well?

A: Some brands of echinacea carry a warning to avoid use if one is pregnant or breastfeeding, so avoid those, even though researchers have found that only trace amounts of echinacea leach into breast milk. If the product label doesn't contain such a warning, it is safe to take echinacea in small doses (e.g., 2 capsules of 450 milligrams, three times a day) for no more than a few days to ward off a cold. However, avoid taking echinacea on a daily basis. In time, your body will build up a tolerance, and then echinacea won't help ward off colds.

Engorged Breasts

Q: My breasts are so engorged that they look like balloons. My newborn can't latch on, or if he does manage, he loses his grip. I tried expressing some milk, but my breasts are still too hard. What can I do?

A: Most new moms have engorged breasts—it's common, but painful. As the milk comes in for the first time, the vessels surrounding the lymph nodes are flushed with blood. Engorged breasts are hard, are hot, can hurt, and—as you pointed out—can make it difficult for a newborn to latch on because the aerola is too firm. There are several ways to relieve engorged breasts:

- Take a very warm (but not unbearably hot) shower. Stand with your back to the shower, and gently massage out the milk by hand. (Don't worry—you'll still have plenty of milk left for the baby, and it will take a while for your breasts to replace the expressed milk.) Express until your breasts are soft enough to allow the baby to latch on and suckle. Your breasts will still feel huge, but more pliant.
- Place raw cabbage leaves—whole or torn—in your bra. No one really knows why this works, but something in the cabbage leaves reduces engorgement.
- Warm a couple of hand towels in the dryer or microwave. (They're ready when they're hot enough to barely handle, like the heated towels that customers use at Japanese restaurants.) Lay the warm towels on your breasts. The heat probably will inspire some letdown, which will relieve the pressure, and the towels will absorb the milk.

- Use a breast pump (electric pumps are better than hand pumps) to empty some milk from your breasts. This is easier than taking a shower if you're still recovering from a c-section, and you can save the milk in the freezer to use later.
- Let the baby nurse as often as she wants. This will help your milk supply stabilize more quickly and reduce the engorgement. Feeding sessions may last 15 to 40 minutes at first. As your baby gets older, she'll become more efficient at nursing and may nurse for only 10 to 15 minutes or so.

Find the number for your local La Leche League club, and call the leader; she can share practical advice and lend support.

See also Breast Compression; Cabbage Leaves and Engorged Breasts; Lactation Consultant; Pumping, About; Appendix

Evening Madness

Q: My 3-month-old daughter is really fussy in the evening. She wants to nurse constantly—every hour, sometimes. At most, she goes 2 or 3 hours between feeds. If she falls asleep nursing, she wakes up again in an hour. Is she getting enough milk?

A: Most babies have a fussy period in the evening. One mom refers to the period between 5 and 7 P.M. as UnHappy Hour. It's a rough time of day—you're exhausted and stressed, ready to start winding down, and preoccupied with dinner plans and other chores, while the baby, still fresh from an afternoon nap, is full of beans. And if she's going through a growth spurt, the demands on you increase dramatically. If you go into the evening expecting her to be cranky, you'll endure it more easily. If she's nursing constantly, she may be nursing as much for comfort as for food.

Is it possible to have someone else assume your late afternoon/early evening duties for a few days, so you and the baby can have 3 hours alone? (Think of it as a short-term nursing holiday.) You'll get a chance to rest, or at least to concentrate on one thing instead of worrying about several.

And if you haven't already established a predictable evening routine, do it now. Set a pattern, and stick to it: nursing, a bath, floor time, cuddle and lullaby/book time, and a bedtime feed. If the baby needs to nurse, let her, but continue with the routine after she's latched off. The routine is as much for your sake as for hers.

Remember: This, too, shall pass. In another month or so, she'll settle down and be able to go longer between feedings.

See also Growth Spurts, About

Excess Lipase

See Lipase, Excess

Exercise and Breastfeeding

Q: I gained well over 30 pounds during pregnancy, and I've lost only half of it so far. (My daughter is nearly 12 weeks old.) I'm breastfeeding, and I intend to nurse as long as she wants. But I've heard that any aerobic sports can adversely affect my milk supply. Is this true? It took me nearly a month until my daughter didn't need supplements in addition to my breast milk.

A: Exercise should not decrease your milk supply. Some studies have shown that anaerobic exercise at maximum intensity can increase the lactic acid content in breast milk.

If you exercise vigorously, it may temporarily change the flavor of your milk (because of the increase in lactic acid), but many babies don't even notice. If yours does, nurse her before you exercise, and wait an hour or so after exercising before nursing again.

One tip: Wear a very supportive exercise bra. Some women use a stretchy exercise bra over the nursing bra for additional support.

Drink plenty of fluids, especially water, to replace what you lose during your workouts.

And don't stress if a few stubborn pounds refuse to slip off.

Some women don't return to their prepregnancy weight until after weaning. Most mothers take an average of $5^1/_2$ months to return to their prepregnancy weight, so it does take time.
See also Running and Breastfeeding; Weight Loss

Expressing by Hand

Q: I need to express about 12 ounces of milk—enough for two or three bottles a day. But I don't want to buy a pump. Can I get away with expressing by hand?
A: If you've got a good supply, an active letdown, and lots of time and patience, you can learn to hand-express as much milk as you need. Some moms find that expressing milk with a manual pump takes only a little more time than with an electric pump.

Another caveat: Potential sanitation problems are the main concern when you're expressing by hand. Unless you express directly into a funnel specifically designed for this purpose (Medela makes one), your milk is more exposed to the air (and any germs in it), and it may trickle down your fingers. You'll need to be meticulous about washing your hands before and after expressing. Being comfortable, confident, and relaxed is the best way to produce and express enough milk.
See also Supply Problems, About

Extended Breastfeeding

Q: I plan to nurse my son, who's 18 months old now, until he self-weans. I don't think it's a big deal, but friends and family members are starting to make comments. What should I tell them?
A: Tell them you're planning to nurse until he self-weans. Humor disarms most critics. One mom claimed that she planned to enroll her son in junior college for the first 2 years so he could come home to nurse. She even had a Top 10 Reasons to Nurse Your College-Age Child:

Better than dorm food
Raises IQ for those tough chemistry exams
Fewer trips to the infirmary
Saves on meal plan bills
Available even when cafeteria is closed
You know where they are, at least during nursing time
Helps them sleep
Instant comfort after sorority or fraternity hazing
Boosts your metabolism at a time of life when it otherwise slows down
No longer necessary to monitor your own alcohol intake, since your child's is probably higher

See also Critics, Coping with

Eye Exams

Q: I've been wearing glasses throughout my pregnancy, which altered my vision so much that I could no longer use my contacts. Now I'm breastfeeding, and I'd love to wear contacts again.

I've heard that opthamologists won't examine your eyes if you're a nursing mom, because of hormone fluctuations, but an optometrist said breastfeeding doesn't have the same impact on prescription changes. Who's right?

A: Pregnancy can temporarily change your vision, but your eyes typically revert back to whatever they were within a few weeks after birth, whether you're breastfeeding or using formula. Cautious doctors might be (needlessly) concerned because they're uncertain what percent of the drops used in eye exams might be leached into breast milk.

Ezzo, Gary

Q: A friend told me I should be breastfeeding my 9-week-old son on the Ezzo schedule—that he'd be sleeping all night, and be a better baby. What is the Ezzo schedule?

A: Gary Ezzo, founder of Growing Families International and its programs, including Preparation for Parenting and Growing Kids God's Way, advocates managing infants through scheduled feedings and strict discipline. His programs, usually taught in churches, and *On Becoming Babywise,* a secular version of the *Preparation for Parenting* class handbook coauthored with a young pediatrician, have reached more than 600,000 people to date.

Most pediatricians and other medical experts are skeptical of Ezzo, who has had no medical training. Several physicians have publicly said that the program he advocates can endanger babies' health. A newborn is most vulnerable to such rigid scheduling.

Early versions of the Ezzo program discouraged feeding babies more frequently than every 3 hours, and some infants required medical attention for dehydration and weight loss. In later editions of his publications, Ezzo revised his recommendations to more closely reflect the American Academy of Pediatrics (AAP) recommendations.

The AAP and its members have expressed concerns with Ezzo's teachings, and recently encouraged pediatricians to closely monitor babies whose parents follow his program. Dr. William Sears and Dr. Marianne Neifert, pediatricians and authors of parenting books, both recommend demand-regulated, not parent-directed, feedings.

For more information and opinions online about Ezzo, "On Becoming Babywise," "Growing Families International," and "Growing Kids God's Way," see the following Web sites online:

http://www.family.com/Features/family__1997__09/minn/minn97ezzo/minn97e
http://www.geocities.com/Heartland/Meadows/3246/brave.html
http://www.bhip.com/features/eqa.htm
http://www.fix.net/~rprewett/fam.html
http://www.fix.net/~rprewett/maynard.html
http://www.geocities.com/Heartland/Meadows/3246/insensitive.html
http://www.fix.net/~rprewett/concerns.html
http://www.rapidnet.com/~jbeard/bdm/exposes/ezzo/

http://www1.gospelcom.net/HyperNews/get/tt/fo0297/20/4/½.html

http://www.mailng-list.net/redrhino/Ezzo/files.html

http://redrhino.mas.vcu.edu/Ezzo/gfiresponse.html

http://redrhino.mas.vcu.edu/Ezzo/moral.html

http://www.fix.net/~rprewett/grace-ezzo.html

See also Scheduled Feedings; Schedules for Feeding and Infant Management Programs, About

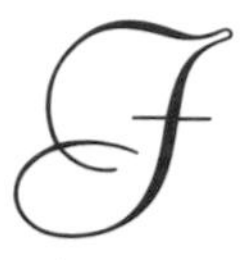

Fathers and Breastfeeding

Q: Ever since our daughter was born 3 weeks ago, my husband feels like a fifth wheel. He's very supportive of breastfeeding, but obviously he can't help with that. What can he do to establish his own special relationship with the baby?

A: Your daughter is lucky to have such a devoted father. Researchers at the University of North Carolina at Chapel Hill found that fathers play a pivotal role in the initial decision to breastfeed as well as increasing its duration. ("Effect of Expectant Mothers' Feeding Plan on Prediction of Fathers' Attitudes Regarding Breastfeeding," *American Journal of Perinatology,* Vol. 10, No. 4, July 1993.)

When the baby is finished nursing, he can burp her or cuddle her to sleep. When she wakes up, he can get her, change her, and bring her to you if she's crying to be fed. Encourage him to focus on playing with the baby—making eye contact, babbling, and playing peek-a-boo.

He can take her on walks, using a stroller or frontpack, or put on some music and dance with her. One dad established own special relationship with his infant son by using the same blanket each time he held the baby—it became the Daddy blankie. They still use it at storytime, now that the baby is a toddler, and it's invaluable when Daddy works late or is gone overnight on business trips.

Feeding-Schedules

See Ezzo, Gary; Scheduled Feedings; Schedules for Feeding and Infant Management Programs, About

Fennel Tea

Q: I've heard that fennel tea can help calm a fussy baby. Is it safe for a 4-month-old baby to have fennel tea?

A: A teaspoon or two of fennel tea may help relieve gastric distress and cramps in babies, but remember: Babies are like adults. Each reacts a little differently. If a couple of teaspoons of fennel tea helps calm your sister's baby, it may have no effect on your son. It won't hurt, either, and the licorice taste alone may be so appealing that your baby forgets to cry for a while. Most babies are fussy between the hours of 5 and 10 P.M.—known as Un-Happy Hour—and nothing except holding them really seems to help. Fussiness that lasts most of the day and night is not normal. It may indicate food allergies and sensitivities, or other problems that require your pediatrician's attention.

See also Allergies (Baby's), About; Allergies, Dairy; Colic; Foods to Avoid

Fenugreek

Q: Will fenugreek boost my milk supply? At the health food store, it's sold as capsules and loose, like tea. Are you supposed to cook fenugreek, or take it like vitamins?

A: Fenugreek, like blessed thistle and some other herbs, enjoys a long-standing reputation as a milk stimulator in lactating women. It's one of the primary ingredients in Mother's Milk Tea, which is how many moms ingest fenugreek, and also in capsules (two capsules, three or four times a day, for 3 to 7 days).

Does fenugreek help improve milk supply? Many nursing moms, lactation consultants, La Leche League leaders, and others swear by fenugreek. But some lactation consultants and doctors are skeptical. No epidemiological studies solidly prove that fenugreek or other herbs do, in fact, increase your milk supply. And many nursing moms are disappointed to find that fenugreek may fail to live up to its advertising. Fenugreek, like other galactogogues, can't fix milk supply problems by itself. You'll need to nurse or pump more frequently, and get help from a breastfeeding expert.

Fenugreek has its downsides: It makes your sweat and urine take on a distinct maple odor, and it can cause gas and diarrhea. *See also Herbal Remedies and Supplements, About; Mother's Milk Tea; Supply Problems, About*

Finger-Feeding

Q: Nurses at the hospital bottle-fed my prematurely born daughter, who had to be on a respirator after a complicated delivery, so she has nipple confusion. Another mom told me that she can learn to nurse again by finger-feeding. How does finger-feeding work?

A: Finger-feeding, also called suck training, teaches babies the proper sucking technique. Ask a lactation consultant experienced in finger-feeding and supplemental nursing system feeding to help you. To finger-feed, you insert your finger as far into your baby's mouth as the nipple would go, back to the spot where the hard palate meets the soft palate (but not farther, or she'll gag). Most babies will reflexively start sucking.

One method of finger-feeding uses surgical tubing threaded along your finger, running past your palm and back to a bottle of expressed milk. You can also use a periodontic syringe, which has a curved plastic tip that slips between the baby's mouth and the finger your baby is sucking. Both techniques reward the baby for sucking by supplying small amounts of milk.

Finger-feeding is simple but extremely time-consuming. A single feeding can last an hour or longer, and within 90 minutes, it's time to begin again. Many lactation experts consider finger-feeding among the most successful techniques to teach breastfeeding to a baby with a poor suck or nipple confusion. A few babies are able to make the transition from finger-feeding to breastfeeding within a few days, but often it takes a week—sometimes longer. You'll need professional help to get the knack of finger-feeding and to make the transition from finger-feeding to breastfeeding.

See also Lactation Consultant; Paladai; Palate, High; Tube Feeding Lactation Aid

Fingers, Sucking While Nursing

Q: My little one keeps sticking his fingers in his mouth when he's nursing. Sometimes he manages to get them in without breaking the latch, so he's sucking his fingers and eating at once. Has this happened to anyone else? Should I worry about this interfering with his nutrition? How can I get him to stop?

A: Well, you don't need to worry about whether he's got a good sucking instinct! Yes, this happens a lot, especially with babies who have a strong need to suck.

It doesn't really affect his caloric intake, but the nipple's owner feels frustrated (and worse if his fingernails are long and sharp). You can try to discourage him by pulling his fingers out of his mouth when he's nursing. Be persistent, and simultaneous finger-sucking and breastfeeding will lose its appeal.

Flailing

Q: My 3-month-old daughter gets so excited to nurse that she flails her little arms and legs around, arches her back, and pulls herself off the breast several times during feedings. It's like trying to nurse a chimpanzee. How can I get her to calm down?

A: Do you have an active letdown reflex? If your milk sprays out when you let down, she may be getting too much milk to swallow. If that's the case, pump or hand-express a little milk before putting her on your breast; that should slow the flow.

If she latches on; sucks a little; and flails, cries, kicks, and generally rejects the breast, she may not be hungry. Some babies tend to eat better in the evening and can go 3 or 4 hours between feeding sessions during the morning and afternoon.

If she seems to be indecisive, or repeatedly pulls on and off, it can be a sign of a yeast infection (is thrush a possibility?) or reflux, which you should check out with her pediatrician.

If she's just an active nurser, consider investing in a nursing pillow (Boppy, My Brest Friend, and Medela all are good choices) to help her feel more secure.

See also Overactive Letdown

Flat Nipples

See Breast Shells; Nipple Shields

Flu, Breastfeeding When You Have

Q: I'm sick with the flu. Can I still breastfeed, or do I have to throw out the milk I've pumped since I got sick? I don't want my 3-month-old son to get the flu, too. Also, my milk supply seems to be decreasing. Will it come back when I get well?

A: You and your son are better off if you continue to breastfeed when you're sick with a cold or flu, or nearly any other illness, including vomiting, diarrhea, and rashes. With some rare exceptions, a mother who's ill should continue to breastfeed. You're infectious several days before you realize that you're sick. By then, the baby's already been exposed, too. (It's also possible that the baby gave you the infection but was symptom free.)

The antibodies in your breast milk will help him fight off the illness and mitigate its severity. Pour yourself a pitcher of water, or water and juice, and get into bed with your baby instead of wasting energy pumping.

Flu Shots

Q: Is it okay to get a flu shot while I'm breastfeeding, or could the vaccine somehow affect my milk?

A: Flu shots won't compromise the safety of your milk—in fact, because the vaccine affords you some protection from the flu, if it prevents you from getting sick, your baby will benefit indirectly. The vaccine's effect on breast milk is negligible—it won't directly provide antibodies through your milk for the baby.

Fluconazole (Diflucan)

Q: My doctor prescribed fluconazole to treat thrush, but he also told me that it will transfer into my milk. Should I continue breastfeeding, or pump and dump until the thrush is resolved?

A: Fluconazole, an antifungal agent that is taken by mouth or intravenously, does leach into breast milk, which actually benefits your baby. Usually, if you have thrush, so does your baby. Fluconazole is being used for babies in the early stages of thrush. So yes, you can continue breastfeeding while you're taking fluconazole.

It may take a few days before you notice a change. Fluconazole will stop—but not kill—the fungus, and *Candida albicans,* which causes thrush, is increasingly resistant to fluconazole. (Less than 10 years ago, a dose of 100 milligrams daily for 10 days eliminated thrush symptoms in most women. By 1999, doctors were prescribing 400 milligrams for the first day, followed by 200 milligrams a day for at least 2 weeks.)

See also Gentian Violet; Thrush, About

Foods to Avoid

Q: Are there certain foods in my diet that cause gas and colic in my baby?

A: Some foods do adversely affect a baby's developing digestive system. Dairy products are the worst culprit—anything made from cow's milk and its by-products, including casein and whey. Start bringing a magnifying glass along to the grocery store, and read product labels.

Eliminate one food at a time for at least 2 weeks. If you notice a difference in your baby's demeanor, you'll know that you've nailed down the offender. Babies who are sensitive to one food, like dairy, may also be sensitive to other foods, so you may need to repeat the cycle a few times.

A teaspoon or two of fennel tea can relieve gastric distress in babies.

The most common foods that cause gas and irritation in babies:

Dairy products, including milk, cheese, ice cream, and cream-based soups
Soy milk and soy bean products
Acidic foods, including tomatoes and tomato products, and citrus fruits
Coffee and soft drinks containing caffeine
Chocolate (it contains theobromide as well as caffeine)
Broccoli and cauliflower
Onions and leeks
Garlic
Some spices, including cinnamon and allspice

Tips on managing a baby who's sensitive or allergic to certain foods:

- Resist the urge to feed your baby the same foods that other babies eat. Don't feel guilty because your baby can't eat certain treats or other foods: She doesn't know the difference, and she won't suffer on a restricted diet as long as her nutritional needs are met.
- If your baby rejects a food, it may be an indication that

she's allergic to it. Children often reject the foods to which they are sensitive. (Sensitivities don't last forever; you can try introducing the food again in a month or so, and watch for any reaction.)

- Always inform caregivers—relatives, friends, babysitters, day care workers—about the child's special requirements. Make their job easier, and your child's health safer, by providing safe foods from home instead of relying on food from other sources.
- Remember that symptoms don't always occur immediately but can be delayed for several hours or even a couple of days. The same time span applies to breastfeeding mothers who eat something to which their babies are allergic.
- Once you've recognized and treated the symptoms, it may take some time before the symptoms clear up. It may be a couple of days or a couple of weeks.

Other references for parents concerned about babies and allergies: *Solving the Puzzle of Your Hard-to-Raise Child* by William G. Crook, MD, and Laura Stevens; *Medications and Mother's Milk* by Thomas W. Hale, MD, and *Is This Your Child?* by Doris Rapp.

See also Colic; Dairy Sensitivities

Football Hold

Q: I'm confident with the football hold, but it's not that convenient now that my son has started kicking the back of the sofa or the headboard, which pulls my nipple. He's only 3 weeks old. How can I teach him to stop this? I can't nurse without supporting my back, and he won't nurse when I try other positions.

A: Have you tried nursing in the side-lying position? Babies who do well with the football hold like lying to nurse, especially if they resist the cradle hold. (Some babies dislike feeling confined.)

If you want to stick with the football hold, you can try sup-

porting your back by positioning a couple of cushions or pillows behind your back, and laying the baby on a nursing pillow next to you, so his feet can't reach the sofa.
See also Positions, About

Foremilk and Hindmilk

Q: How can I tell if my 2-week-old baby's getting enough hindmilk? I sense that he's getting mostly foremilk, because he seems hungry just a short time after nursing. He's an erratic nurser—he latches on for a few minutes, nurses vigorously, and then latches off even though there's still so much milk in my breasts that it literally drips out.

A: Foremilk is the watery milk, relatively low in fat, that the baby gets when he first latches on. The letdown reflex triggers your breasts to release fat globules into your milk, turning it into the high-fat hindmilk. There's a significant fat difference between foremilk and hindmilk: Foremilk is only about 2 percent fat, while hindmilk is often 10 percent or more fat. The increased fat satiates a nursing baby. The letdown reflex also triggers your other breast to start releasing fat, so when you switch breasts during a feed, your baby will immediately get a combination of foremilk and hindmilk.

You can tell if your baby's getting enough hindmilk by checking his stools. If they're mustard-colored, he's getting enough milk—he's just an efficient nurser. If they're green-tinted, especially if they're bright green, then he's not getting enough hindmilk. (Babies who don't get enough hindmilk also tend to be cranky. A foremilk-heavy diet leaves them gassy and hungry.)

Some newborns tend to cluster-nurse: They breastfeed energetically but for short periods (less than 10 minutes) and want to nurse again in 60 to 90 minutes. It's exhausting for you, as a new mom, but it's not unusual as babies settle into their feeding and sleeping cycles. Breast compression may help fill him up a little more.

It may be helpful to take a nursing holiday—a few days or a

weekend when you do nothing but stay in bed (or on the sofa) with the baby, some good paperback books or videos, and nurse, nurse, nurse.

See also Allergies; Foods to Avoid; Colic; Stools, Green

Formula, About

Breast milk is best for your baby, as even the formula companies acknowledge. If you choose to use formula to supplement or replace your own milk, it's smart to take some precautions. Record the lot numbers (on the label) of all formula you use. This information is crucial if your child becomes ill: It's possible for formula itself to cause an illness.

When you're mixing formula, use the measuring scoop that's provided in the can, and measure exactly. Too much or too little can make your baby ill. Use distilled water or cold water—never well water or tap water from old plumbing—to make formula, and boil it before adding it to the formula. (If you are traveling, use bottled water or a water filter capable of removing *Giardia* and other microorganisms.)

Start with a dairy-based formula, unless you have a family history of dairy allergies, and start with the smallest size available. You may need to try several kinds of formula before you find one that your baby will like or tolerate. (Avoid using homemade formula, soy milk or soy-based drinks, rice milk, or other alternatives; they lack the nutrients your baby needs, and may make your baby ill.) Signs of a potential formula intolerance are spitting up frequently, choking, colic, a skin rash, or consistent nasal congestion.

Babies who cannot tolerate any formula, and who display signs of failure to thrive or other disorders, may qualify for donor milk from a mother's milk bank.

If your baby is 4 months old or younger, boil everything you use to feed the baby—bottles, nipples, etc.—after each feeding to sterilize the equipment. If you use disposable bottles (plastic bags), take care to avoid touching the interior of the bag.

Never microwave formula to heat it. A bottle can develop hot spots that may burn and injure your baby's mouth.

Never prop a bottle. Propping can cause dental problems, including caries. When you're giving a bottle, alternate the arm you use to hold the baby; this is more stimulating for the baby than to hold him in the same position each time.

Check the nipple each time you prepare a bottle. If the nipple is cracked or split, throw it away.

Refrigerate premixed formula and cans of powdered formula to discourage bacteria and contamination. Unused or leftover formula must be thrown out within half an hour. After that, bacteria levels are unsafe. Formula-fed babies tend to be gassy, and they need to be burped often during a feeding. Their stools are more dense than a breastfed baby's stools.

Formula, Supplementing with

Q: My sister-in-law told me that if I supplement with formula, it will cause problems for my 6-month-old baby. I can't pump enough to give my day-care provider as much breast milk as she needs. Is it so bad to use formula to make up the difference?

A: If you're exclusively breastfeeding your baby, you usually don't need formula. But it can be difficult to pump enough to satisfy a growing baby, especially during growth spurts, if you're working too. Your baby can safely take both breast milk and formula. The only concern might be that if your baby is less than 6 weeks old, she could be susceptible to nipple confusion and find that bottle-feeding is easier than breastfeeding.

Look at it this way: At least your baby's had the advantage of a breast milk–only diet for 6 months. That's longer than many moms manage! And if you continue to nurse when you're with the baby, she'll still get the immunological and nutritional benefits of breast milk.

See also Formula, About; Formula vs. Breast Milk; Nipple Confusion

Formula vs. Breast Milk

Q: My mom used formula for me and my three brothers. She insists that it's better than breast milk. I've read that breastfed babies are less at risk for ear infections and other illnesses. Is that true?

A: As a group, breastfed babies tend to have lower rates of certain illnesses than do formula-fed babies. There have been hundreds of clinical studies, with results published in epidemiological journals, contrasting breastfed and formula-fed babies. Overwhelmingly, those studies found that breastfed babies are less at risk for ear infections, pneumonia, gastroenteritis, necrotizing entercolitis, Crohn's disease, allergies, asthma, childhood and adult cancers, diabetes, obesity, and heart disease. (That's why formula companies include a packaging disclaimer acknowledging that breast milk is superior to their product.)

This does not mean that breastfed babies aren't susceptible to those diseases. It means they have a better chance of resisting them, thanks to the antibodies associated with breast milk.

Formula is an incomplete attempt to copy breast milk. Formulas contain no antibodies, living cells, enzymes, or hormones. The fats and proteins in breast milk are markedly different from those in formula. Breast milk is custom-made in response to your baby's health and dietary needs, but formula is one-size-fits-all. And, because babies don't absorb nutrients from formula as efficiently as they do from breast milk, formula contains far more protein, aluminum, iron, cadmium, and manganese than does breast milk—which sounds like an advantage, until you learn that the extra supplements generally are excreted. Infant formula is better for babies than cow's milk, goat's milk, or adult formulas (nutritional supplements), all of which can cause enormous problems in babies.

So: Breast milk is better than formula, especially for newborns. Some babies can't tolerate formula, and it is frustrating—sometimes impossible—to find an artificial human milk that they can take. (An alternative: donor milk from human milk banks.)

See also Formula, About; Milk Banks; Appendix

Frantic Nurser

Q: My 6-month-old is a champion air-gulper, even when he has a good latch-on. He thrashes when he's first put to the breast. He seems to be so frantic to eat that he can't just nurse calmly. Then he pulls and thrashes so much I have to burp him three or four times in the middle of a feed. How can I get him to slow down?

A: It might help to give him something to suck on until he's less overexcited about sucking and calm enough to nurse. You can try letting him suck on your pinky finger for a minute or so, and see if that helps him settle a bit.

How's your letdown? Does your milk spray out when you start nursing, or when the baby pulls off your nipple? He may be reacting to an overactive letdown that makes it difficult for him to keep up with the flow.

Conversely, if your flow is slow when your son thrashes around, he may be trying to get more milk. (In that case, try breast compression.)

Could he be teething? Have you tried giving him a frozen washcloth or a biter biscuit (teething biscuit) to gnaw on before offering your breast? The combination of a new taste and texture may be enough to calm him so he can concentrate on nursing.

See also Breast Compression; Colic; Growth Spurts, About; Overactive Letdown

Frozen Expressed Milk with Odd Smell

Q: When I defrosted some breast milk from my freezer, I noticed that it had a strange smell. It isn't sour and doesn't seem to be off—I tasted it, and it tastes OK. But it definitely smells different. Should I use it or toss it?

A: When breast milk is frozen, one of the enzymes in it breaks down, causing the milk to take on a sort of soapy smell. It can be so subtle that some women never notice it. As long as the milk tastes fresh (sample a drop or two to be sure), and you know it's not sour, it's OK to give to your baby.

If it tastes and smells bad when you've just expressed it, that's another story. It may be a sign of excess lipase, which can cause expressed milk to go bad within 2 or 3 hours.
See also Lipase, Excess; Pumping, About

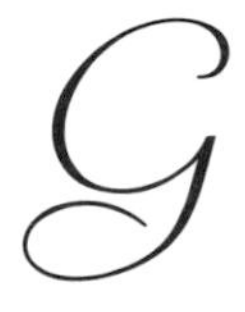

Galactorrhea

Q: Is it common to be able to express milk for a long time, even after weaning? I weaned my older daughter 2 months ago, and sometimes I still find damp spots on my bra.

A: Some women, especially those whose milk supply was abundant while they were nursing, continue to produce milk for months, and sometimes years, after weaning. Some women can express a drop of milk as they're entering menopause.

Gas, Burping

Q: My 3-week-old son burps only about half the time after feedings. Either he burps within a couple of minutes, or not at all. If he doesn't burp, I try patting him for 10 minutes, sitting him up, putting him on my knee, but—nothing. Then he wakes up about an hour later with lots of gas. What am I doing wrong?

A: Sounds as if he may not always have a good seal when he's nursing. If you have an abundant milk supply, he could easily nurse for a full feeding, even without a good seal, and be gulping extra air as he nurses. Dimpling cheeks, or making loud smacking or clicking sounds as he nurses, are signs that he's not sealing well.

Try feeding him more frequently, so he takes in less milk at each feed. Express a little milk before offering your breast, and try feeding him on only one breast at each nursing session. Make sure he's positioned and properly latched on.

After nursing him during the daytime, hold him upright instead of laying him down after a feed. Babies between 2 and 12 weeks old tend to be gassy, and nobody really knows why. He may be easier to burp when he's older. Rest as much as you can, and eat well. By taking care of yourself, you'll be able to take the best care of your baby.

See also Burping a Sleepy Baby; Colic; Latching On, About; Positions, About

Gastroesophageal Reflux

See Reflux

Gentian Violet

Q: I have thrush, and a friend told me to try gentian violet. What is it? Do I use it just on my thrush, or does the baby use it, too?

A: Gentian violet, sold at most health food stores, is a dye in a 1 percent alcohol solution, used to treat a thrush infection of both mother and baby. Thrush is a yeast infection *(Candida albicans)*, which usually shows up as white patches in a baby's mouth or as a diaper rash. A nursing mother with thrush has sore nipples and often shooting pains in her breasts.

Be careful when you use gentian violet: It is messy, it stains permanently, and it can stain again even after it dries if it gets wet. (Rubbing alcohol can help lighten the stains.) Wear old clothes during the 3-day course of treatment.

To use gentian violet on your baby, dip a cotton swab in water and then into the bottle of gentian violet. Slip the swab into your baby's mouth and let her suck on it for a few seconds to distribute the gentian violet around her mouth. If she won't suck the swab, paint the inside of her mouth and get as much solution as possible on her tongue and the inside of her cheeks.

To use it on yourself, dip a cotton swab directly in the gentian violet and paint your nipples with it. If your nipples are extremely sore, dip the swab in water first to mitigate the alcohol's sting.

Treat the baby's mouth and your nipples once a day for 3 days. You should notice some relief after the first treatment, and the pain should be gone by the third day. If it's not, see your doctor.

Make sure that all objects that go into your baby's mouth—pacifiers, toys, artificial nipples—are boiled each day for at least 20 minutes. If you use a breast pump, boil the parts once a day for 20 minutes.

If your baby has a yeast diaper rash, launder her cloth diapers and clothing as usual, and add a cup of vinegar (per load) to an extra rinse cycle. Wash your own bras in hot soapy water and hang them in the sunlight to dry.

See Thrush, About

Goldenseal

Q: I used to take goldenseal every day as a dietary supplement. Now that I'm breastfeeding, I need to know if goldenseal will leach into my milk to benefit my baby.

A: Goldenseal can leach into your milk, but it may do your baby more harm than good. Goldenseal should not be taken daily by anyone, and especially not by a breastfeeding mother. Extended use of goldenseal can deplete your body's levels of some B vitamins, and it can also cause an imbalance in the healthy intestinal flora.

Green Breast Milk

Q: I expressed some breast milk today, and I was shocked when the milk that I pumped was light green! I nearly fell over. I didn't notice its color when I nursed my 4-month-old earlier. It doesn't seem to bother her. None of my breastfeeding friends have ever heard of this. Should I toss out the expressed milk?

A: Green breast milk is unusual, but it won't harm your baby.

Often green-tinged milk is caused by overindulging in iron supplements, soft drinks (including Gatorade) colored with aggressive dyes, and even overloading on asparagus and certain other green vegetables. Have you had a plugged duct or a breast infection? Sometimes greenish or yellowish milk emerges when a plugged duct opens up.

Your milk should revert to its normal color within 24 hours. The color doesn't affect the milk, although if the culprit was asparagus, your daughter might have noticed a difference in the milk's taste. There's no need to pump and dump, but you probably should cut back on the iron supplements, soft drinks, or asparagus.

See also Breast Infections; Plugged Ducts, About

Green Stools

See Stools, Green

Growth Charts

Q: My mother-in-law thinks my 7-month-old daughter is underweight. The pediatrician isn't concerned because she nurses at least five times a day and eats lots of solids. But according to the official growth chart, my daughter is in the 70th percentile, lengthwise, and below the 20th percentile in weight. I know the growth chart is based on formula-fed babies. Is there a growth chart for breastfed babies?

A: You're right: Most pediatricians use growth charts whose standards are based on formula-fed babies. Both formula-fed babies and breastfed babies share the same growth patterns for the first 3 months, but after that, things change. Generally, by age 1, a breastfed baby is long and lean, and a formula-fed baby is chubby.

The World Health Organization recently published a growth chart that specifically evaluates breastfed babies. So far, the data are still being collected, so the chart is being used by researchers rather than pediatricians' offices. However, because the WHO is aggressively promoting breastfeeding, the new charts, which are based on a more equable sampling and distribution of breastfed and formula-fed babies, should be available soon in the United States.

Maybe your mother-in-law can accompany you on your next visit to the pediatrician, and your doctor can reassure her fears. All babies grow at different rates. How much a baby weighs, or how long or tall she is, matters less than whether her weight gain and growth are consistent.

See also Weight and Growth Charts, About

Growth Spurts, About

Most growth spurts last 2 or 3 days, sometimes a little longer. Babies seem to hit growth spurts at between 2.5 and 5 weeks, 6 and 7 weeks, 12 and 13 weeks, and every 2 months or so afterward. (Babies also want to nurse a lot when they're teething, or when they're at the edge of a developmental milestone, e.g., sitting up, crawling, pulling up, or walking.)

During a growth spurt, a baby needs more milk and will nurse more spontaneously and more often, and take longer than usual at the breast. You'll know that your baby's hit a growth spurt when your day is consumed by breastfeeding—and whenever you're not breastfeeding, you've just finished a feed or are about to be summoned to another. It's a lot like cluster feeding, when a newborn nurses every half hour or so for several hours.

Growth spurts can be exhausting and frustrating for moms. During a growth spurt, anything resembling a regular schedule is thrown off—and that includes babies who usually sleep and eat at predictable intervals. You might feel defensive when people ask why the baby's nursing so often, or suggest supplementing with formula. Don't resign yourself to using formula if you're determined to breastfeed exclusively—your body responds to the baby's needs by making more milk, and supplementing will only throw your milk supply off balance.

If you have a stash of expressed milk, you can buy yourself some time by giving the baby a bottle or sippy cup with 4 or 5 ounces of expressed milk. (Caveat: She may refuse to take milk from a bottle, especially if you're the one offering it. Breastfed babies usually prefer to get their milk directly from the source.)

Avoid the temptation to count how many times your baby is nursing, or how long she's nursing—growth spurts tend to throw routines and schedules out the window. It's not unusual for a baby to embark on a nursing marathon all evening, or in the middle of the night, when she's in the midst of a growth spurt. Be patient. This, too, will pass. Meanwhile, turn a blind eye to the housework and call out for pizza.

Growth Spurts, Duration of

Q: My daughter, almost 5 weeks old, suddenly has started nursing around the clock. My mother thinks she's having a growth spurt, and my mother-in-law thinks I'm spoiling her by letting her nurse so often. I don't know who to believe, but I'm not getting anything else done. How long will this last?

A: Growth spurts rarely last longer than 72 hours. (It just seems longer!) During a growth spurt, the baby needs to nurse more often because she needs more calories. You're not spoiling the baby by nursing her on demand—you're meeting her needs.

See also Growth Spurts, About

Grunting While Nursing

Q: My 10-day-old is constantly grunting. She grunts when she's hungry, and after nursing when she's not hungry, and sometimes even in her sleep when she looks as if she's nursing. Is she reacting to something I ate?

A: Have you been nursing her while you're watching *Babe* on video? (Just kidding.)

Does she seem comfortable? Is she gaining appropriately? Does she produce the requisite number of wet and poopy diapers? If she does, you can relax. But if she seems to be grunting to help herself breathe, have your pediatrician see her immediately.

H

Hair, Losing

Q: Breastfeeding is great, now that my 3-month-old and I have conquered his latch-on problems and weathered a couple of plugged ducts. But now my hair is falling out. A good friend who also nurses her baby, a little younger than mine, is having the same problem. Does breastfeeding make your hair fall out?

A: Not directly. A lot of moms lose hair during the postpartum period, especially women whose hair thrived during pregnancy. The same hormones that made your hair thick and glossy are dwindling back to normal levels—and so is your hair.

Eventually, the hair loss will stop, and your hair will look—more or less, so to speak—the way it did before you were pregnant.

Hair on Breasts and Nipples

Q: I have hair around my breast and nipples. Will this affect breastfeeding? Should I have it removed before I have the baby?

A: It is not unusual for women to have some hair on their breasts. Often women with darker complexions have heavier and coarser hair growth than those with a more fair complexion. This will not affect your ability to nurse your baby. It is not necessary to remove it.

Hates to Breastfeed

See Allergies (Baby's), About; Arching Baby; Colic; Discouragement, Dealing with; Overactive Letdown; Pulling on Nipple

Headaches During Letdown

Q: After my milk came in, I've had moderate to killer headaches. At first, I thought they were spinal headaches caused by the epidural, but that's been ruled out. Does this go on as long as I breastfeed? What can I do about it?

A: Some women get painful headaches, and even a mild fever, when their milk first comes in. If your blood pressure is on the high side of normal, the combination of postpartum stress and adjusting to a new baby can send your blood pressure high enough to cause a headache. Even if your blood pressure is normal, the lack of sleep combined with new milk coming in can be agonizing.

The headaches will go away in a few days to a week; you're not doomed to suffer them throughout breastfeeding. Meanwhile, ibuprofen will help numb the headaches.

If you have other children, this is the time for a visit with grandparents or to hire a babysitter—or work out a trade with another mom—to minimize your own stress.

Herbal Remedies and Supplements, About

Many nursing mothers worry about whether they're producing enough milk. The general rule: If you're drinking enough water, juice, or other nonalcoholic fluids (8 to 12 ounces an hour), resting (such as you can), and nursing on demand, your breasts respond by making as much milk as your baby needs. If you're still concerned about boosting your milk supply, lots of nursing mothers swear by certain herbs—fenugreek, blessed thistle, and other herbs—to boost their milk supply, fight colds, and combat other problems. Often these herbs are in the form of teas, so it's hard to say whether a woman's milk supply is enhanced by the herbs or by the additional fluids she's drinking.

Do herbs work? The jury's still out. No medical studies prove the effectiveness of herbal milk-boosters. However, most cultures throughout the world identify certain herbs and plants as galactagogues. Some mothers and doctors believe that herbal remedies are largely responsible for their success in breastfeeding. Other moms report little measurable difference.

Some prescription drugs, as a side effect, do increase milk supply, so it's reasonable to believe that some herbs and plants contain similar chemicals.

However, even herbs and plants have side effects: A drug from what you think of as a "natural" source can be harmful or can have dangerous side effects. (And because herbal supplements are not tightly regulated in the United States, as they are in Germany and some other countries, the herbs used may be contaminated during preparation.) Even though your baby gets only a fraction of the dose you take, with certain herbs and plants, that may be too much for her immature digestive system. St. John's wort, a popular herbal alternative to prescription antidepressants, is not recommended for nursing mothers, partly because of its potential effect on babies.

Fenugreek, blessed thistle, raspberry leaf, fennel, and brewer's yeast are the safe herbal and over-the-counter treatments that seem to successfully increase milk supply. Many natural food stores carry Mother's Milk Tea, which combines those herbs. You can also take them in capsule form, but if you use tea infusions, you'll get the benefit of both fluid and herb.

It is difficult to drink enough tea to make a difference; tinctures and capsules are better. A typical dosage for fenugreek capsules or blessed thistle capsules is two capsules, three or four times a day, for a week. You can also take fenugreek or blessed thistle, or a combination, as a tincture if you don't mind ingesting the tincture's tiny amount of alcohol (which is the reason for the disclaimer that nursing mothers shouldn't take it).

Remember: Herbs or drugs alone probably won't solve the problem. You need to seek help from a lactation consultant to address other possible causes of your difficulties.

See also Antidepressants and Breastfeeding; Fenugreek; Mother's Milk Tea

Herbs to Avoid While Nursing

Q: I usually drink a lot of herbal tea, and I take herbal supplements for energy boost, but a friend told me that I shouldn't be drinking peppermint tea or taking gingko if I'm nursing. Why not?

A: Herbalists say that certain herbs, particularly those in the mint family, can diminish your milk supply. Some doctors and lactation consultants are skeptical about that claim, but they're also skeptical about the claim that herbs can boost your milk supply. Still, if you're having supply problems, and you typically use a lot of herbs in your diet, it's better to be safe than sorry.

Among the other milk-drying suspects: Aloe, alder buckthorn, barberry, cascara sagrada, gingseng, ephedra, ginger, goldenseal, green tea, guarana, kola nut, ma huang, male fern, parsley, purging buckthorn, rhubarb, sage, senna, wormwood, and yerba mate.

High Palate

See Palate, High

Hindmilk, Assessing

See Foremilk and Hindmilk; Stools, Green

HIV and Breast Milk

Q: My day care provider won't give my 6-month-old daughter expressed breast milk because there is a risk that she or the other children at the center will get AIDS. First I was shocked. Then I offered to take a test and prove that I don't carry HIV. She refused. I'm furious. What can I do?

A: It is true that HIV, the virus that causes AIDS, is present in the breast milk of women who are HIV positive. That's why moms in developing countries, particularly those hardest hit by AIDS, are discouraged from breastfeeding. However, the risk of getting HIV from breast milk by handling it is negligible.

HIV is as fragile as it is dangerous. It cannot survive outside the body for more than a few minutes. Contact with air kills the virus.

So your provider is wrong. She may change her mind if you can provide her with research. If she doesn't, your choices are limited. Is her site convenient to your workplace? Could you arrange to come and nurse at feeding times?

If not, and if you want to avoid using formula, your only alternative is to find a breastfeeding-friendly day care provider. The local La Leche League may know of some providers in your area.

Hot Weather and Nursing

Q: It's so hot that the baby and I sweat buckets when we nurse. Is there anything we can do to stay cool at dinner time?

A: Breastfeeding involves so much skin-on-skin contact that it can be problematic when temperatures soar. There are a few tricks to keep sweating to a minimum:

- Lie side by side, instead of holding the baby.
- Wet a towel with cool water, lay the wet towel on your lap, and rest the baby on it.
- Nurse while you're both relaxing in a bath of lukewarm water; you'll feel cooler. (Remember that babies, especially newborns, often urinate or poop while they're nursing. Be prepared to hose down the tub and yourself.)
- Dress minimally. The baby will be fine in just a diaper, and you can wear light, gauzy cotton.

Drink plenty of fluids, especially water, to avoid becoming dehydrated. The baby will nurse as often as she needs, so feed her on demand to keep her well hydrated. (There's no need to supplement with water.)

See also Dehydration; Water Supplements

Hunger, Incessant

Q: My 9-week-old daughter just decided that she needs to eat every hour, or more often. She generally nurses for 20 minutes (10 to 15 minutes on one breast, then topping off on the other), and then drops off to sleep. Almost exactly an hour later, she wakes up again and starts rooting around, sucking on her fist, and wailing her "hungry cry." Before this, she went 2 or 3 hours between feedings. Any suggestions on how to get her to last longer between feedings?

A: Your daughter's about the right age to be going through a growth spurt. During a growth spurt, a baby needs more milk, and in order to get your body to produce enough milk, she needs to nurse frequently for a few days to a week. Once your milk supply matches her need, she'll return to her normal nursing schedule.

See also Growth Spurts, About

Hunger, Judging

Q: Yesterday, my 3-month-old baby started crying to be fed only 30 minutes after I nursed her. I can't believe she's hungry again in such a short time! I know breast milk digests quickly—but that fast? Should I let her cry, or feed her? Could she actually be hungry again so soon?

A: Is she going through a growth spurt? Babies need to eat more, and more frequently, when they're going through a physical or developmental change, like learning a new skill (holding up her head, sitting up, standing, rolling over, etc.).

Babies also need to nurse more frequently when the weather

is especially hot and dry, so they can stay hydrated.

When you're nursing, it's hard to tell how much she's taken in. When you're feeding a baby with a bottle, it's easy to judge how much she's taken in. But lactating breasts are never really empty. The only way to truly judge how much breast milk a baby takes in is to weigh her before and after a feed—a tedious task that is rarely necessary with healthy babies.

I

Immunizations

Q: I need to be immunized for hepatitis B. Will this harm my baby? Do I need to stop breastfeeding until the vaccine leaves my bloodstream?

A: Mothers who receive immunizations (tetanus, rubella, hepatitis B, hepatitis A, etc.) can continue breastfeeding. The vaccines present no risk to the baby and may even benefit her. The sole exception: Babies with compromised immune systems (e.g., HIV-positive babies, and babies with chronic illnesses or congenital infections). Their mothers should not receive immunizations, especially if the baby is being fed formula, because even a weakened live virus presents a hazard to a baby with an immune deficiency.

Imodium (Antidiarrheal)

Q: I have Crohn's disease, and I am prone to diarrhea. I stopped using Imodium after my daughter, now 2 months old, was born, because I worried that it would leach into my breast milk. Is it safe for a nursing mom to take Imodium?

A: Extremely small amounts of Imodium (loperamide) are excreted into breast milk, according to Thomas Hale's *Medica-*

tions and Mothers' Milk, the definitive reference for nursing moms. A breastfed baby who daily consumes 165 milliliters of breast milk per kilogram (about 2.5 ounces per pound) would take in 2,000 times less than the recommended daily dose of Imodium. In other words, you can safely take Imodium.

However, Hale also advises you to watch your baby for abnormally pale skin, increased pulse rate, and constipation. A breastfed baby who is 6 weeks old or older typically has one regular, substantial bowel movement a day (or every day or two) instead of four or more a day, as newborns do. Remember, it's not unusual for a healthy breastfed baby 3 months old or older to go more than a week between (fairly sizable) bowel movements. Small, hard, dry bowel movements indicate constipation.

See also Constipation; Diarrhea, Mother's

Implants, Breast

See Breast Implants

Infection, Breast

See Mastitis, About; Plugged Ducts, About

Insomnia and Nursing

Q: Even though I'm exhausted, I can't sleep when I want to. Instead, I lie in bed, waiting for our month-old baby to wake and want to nurse, or thinking about the things I need to do—including get some sleep! I feel as if I'm sleepwalking. What should I do?

A: Welcome to the club: Anxiety tends to go arm-in-arm with parenthood.

It's possible that your insomnia is diet-related. Sometimes, new mothers can't sleep because they're not eating enough calories. Try to eat some protein an hour or so before going to bed.

Some moms find that their sleep improves when they drink some sweetened warm milk. You can also try taking cat naps—sit down or lie down whenever you get a chance to rest. Instead of worrying about trying to go to sleep, put on some favorite music, close your eyes, and listen for a few minutes.

Exercise can help, too. Try to get out of the house at least once a day and go for a walk (with the baby or alone) in your neighborhood or, if the weather's inclement, at an indoor mall. Yoga and meditation can help you train your brain to calm down and turn off when you need to rest.

Inverted Nipples

See Nipples, Inverted

Iron Supplements

Q: My pediatrician wants me to give my newborn son vitamin D and liquid iron-fortified vitamin supplements. I've heard that breast milk doesn't have as much iron as formula, but is it really necessary to give a new baby vitamins?

A: With the exception of vitamin K, which is given immediately at birth, the current American Academy of Pediatrics recommendation for healthy, full-term breastfed babies is that neither vitamins nor fluoride supplements are necessary until the baby is at least 6 months old. Some doctors who haven't kept up still routinely prescribe supplements, either because they always have prescribed them or because they figure the supplements can't hurt. Studies have shown that supplemental vitamins and iron can interfere with the absorption of the vitamins in breast milk. Healthy infants are born with iron stores, and they rarely need supplemental iron until they're at least 6 months old.

There are exceptions: some prematurely born babies, babies of severely malnourished mothers, or mothers and babies who get little or no sunlight to make vitamin D (particularly if they're dark-skinned), for example. When you're in doubt, a baby's needs should be evaluated on an individual basis.

And if you are advised to use iron supplements, think twice. Unless your hematocrit levels are low (have your doctor check if you suspect you're anemic), a multivitamin will meet your daily needs.

See also Prenatal Vitamins; Vitamin K

IUD, Copper

Q: Now that my child is 2 months old, I need to go back on birth control. Would a copper IUD affect my milk in any way?

A: Unlike intrauterine devices that contain hormones, a copper IUD has no effect on breastfeeding. Like other IUDs, the copper version helps prevent pregnancy . Copper IUDs are effective, long-term, reversible, and reliable—only 8 of 1,000 women using copper IUDs become pregnant during the first year after the IUDs were implanted.

A copper IUD works by releasing copper, interrupting your normal reproductive cycle and causing the endometrium (the lining of the uterus) to shed more often than normal. Side effects often include cramping and a higher risk of anemia caused by irregular and heavy menstrual bleeding. One benefit for breastfeeding moms: They experience less pain during insertion, and are less likely to want a copper IUD removed because of bleeding or pain, than nonlactating women.

See also Birth Control, About

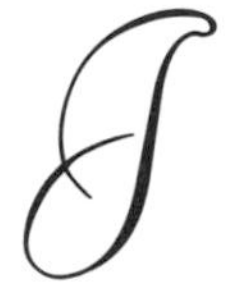

Jaundice, Breast Milk

Q: I thought breast milk was supposed to be best for babies. My pediatrician wants me to put the baby on formula because she says breast milk is causing my newborn's jaundice. How can my breast milk be bad for my baby?

A: There is a condition called breast milk jaundice, but nobody knows exactly what causes it. Breast milk jaundice occurs in 1 in 250 babies. Usually, jaundice is diagnosed in a baby between 5 and 7 days old. It's a common condition—40 percent of babies are diagnosed with some form of jaundice.

Jaundice is caused by a buildup of bilirubin in the baby's blood as the newborn's liver—whose job during pregnancy was handled by the mother—starts functioning on its own. Jaundice usually is resolved within a few days, with phototherapy.

Breast milk jaundice peaks between 10 and 21 days after birth and can last until 4 to 6 weeks after birth.

One way to diagnose breast milk jaundice is to temporarily wean the baby. If the condition is indeed breast milk jaundice, the bilirubin levels will drop in 12 to 24 hours. The levels rise again when the baby resumes nursing, although that's not really a problem—breast milk jaundice does not endanger the baby. Many pediatricians are recommending against temporary weaning as a diagnostic tool for breast milk jaundice, because it can lead to nipple confusion and to formula use by mothers who are groundlessly afraid that their babies will be harmed somehow if they continue nursing.

It is rarely necessary to stop breastfeeding a baby with breast milk jaundice. The jaundice resolves itself, even if you continue to breastfeed. Nipple confusion at this age is a real possibility. You may want to ask another pediatrician for a second opinion.

There are only two known medical conditions that may

require weaning a baby from breast milk. In the first, the baby cannot process the amino acid phenylalinine. The phenylalinine builds up in the baby's body and can lead to serious developmental disabilities. However, the amount of phenylalinine can be calculated, and the baby's blood levels monitored, if you wish to continue breastfeeding. (It means extra work, but if you're determined, you can continue nursing.)

The other condition, which at this point does require weaning, is galactosemia, wherein the baby cannot process galactose, one of the components in lactose.

Newborns are tested for both conditions during the first few days after birth.

See also Nipple Confusion; Pumping, About

Jaundice Won't Go Away

Q: My daughter is nearly a month old and has been exclusively breastfed. She sleeps well and produces lots of wet and poopy diapers, but still has signs of jaundice. Her eyeballs are still yellow. I'm a little freaked out. Am I worrying too much?

A: Normally, newborn jaundice can last 4 to 6 weeks, so the lingering symptoms in your daughter's case may not be cause for worry. However, it is critical to determine the type of bilirubin and to make sure that it is not caused by liver disease. The only way to tell is through blood tests.

Go back to your pediatrician and express your concerns. She can order urine or blood tests to rule out liver disease or other conditions. (The urine test is very simple—it detects the presence of bilirubin in the urine, a sign that the jaundice needs further investigation.)

Other possible signs of liver problems:

- Urine color: Is your daughter's urine clear or yellow?
- Attentiveness: Is she alert or drowsy?
- Unexplained bleeding (e.g., from the nose or umbilical cord).

- Weight gain: Is she losing weight, or gaining only very slowly?
- Unexplained bruises.
- Swollen abdomen.
- Bowel movement color: If they're pale, see a doctor immediately.

Jury Duty

Q: I've just been called for jury duty. My daughter is 3 months old, and she's still breastfed. I do work part time, but I go to her day care provider's to nurse her. Can a juror take breastfeeding breaks?

A: Have you called the registration number listed on your jury duty notice? Many jurisdictions exempt nursing moms from jury duty. (Often, jury duty will be excused or postponed if you're the primary caretaker of a baby or young child.)

You can also present the court with information about contacting the local La Leche League, which is what one breastfeeding mother did when she was summoned to jury duty. The league's area professional liaison responded by providing the judge with the La Leche League's legal packet on jury duty, and information from the American Academy of Pediatrics and other organizations. The mother was excused.

K

K, Vitamin

See Vitamin K

Keflex

See Mastitis, About

L

La Leche League

Q: I would like to join a La Leche League group, but there's no listing in our phone book. How do I get in touch with them?

A: Call 1-800-LALECHE, and ask for contacts in your area. The La Leche League also has a Web site, where you can find answers to frequently asked questions and links to other breastfeeding sites.

Like other organizations with local affiliates, each La Leche League group tends to have a different personality. League members often are stereotyped as hard-core breastfeeding fanatics, and there's more than a grain of truth in that perception, though some groups are more mainstream than others. (It almost goes without saying that LLL groups are pro-breastfeeding, and that moms who use supplemental formula often feel unwelcome.) Individually, members tend to be more flexible. This is a group that you definitely want on your side if you're ever hassled for nursing in public, and it can be a valuable resource if you need someone who can deftly illustrate the right and wrong of different nursing positions. It's worth joining a LLL group just for access to its extensive library and the connections to breastfeeding-friendly pediatricians, restaurants, and other families. If your extended family lives in a distant state, a LLL friend can be invaluable for the late-night help, reassurance, and encouragement that most new moms desperately need.

The La Leche League does not require you to be a member in order to join its meetings, but you must join in order to check out books from its library. Membership costs about $30, which includes a subscription to the organization's magazine, *New Beginnings,* and discounts. The rest of the money pays for printed materials and operating funds.

See Appendix

Lactation Consultant

Q: At the hospital where I delivered my son, a staff lactation consultant breezed in and out of the room. Then, I was so dazed from labor and so new to nursing that I didn't even know what to ask. Now I'm full of questions. How can I find a lactation consultant who'll be helpful?

A: Sounds like you had a bad experience in the hospital. (A lot of hospital lactation consultants are overbooked.)

Start your search by looking for a lactation consultant accredited by the International Board Certified Lactation Consultants.

If you have Internet access, you can track down certified lactation consultants in your area by e-mailing ilca@erols.com and asking for the names of members in your region. (You can also post a question on one of the Internet breastfeeding support newsgroups—such as misc.kids.breastfeeding, or alt.support.breastfeeding—to ask about good lactation consultants in your region.)

Other good sources: Your midwife, pediatrician, or obstetrician/gynecologist, and the local La Leche League. Usually, they know of local lactation consultants. So do business owners who sell or rent breast pumps; many of them also are members of ILCA.

Human milk banks are another possible source. Even if the closest milk bank is several states away, the staffers usually can recommend knowledgeable lactation consultants near you. (Milk banks frequently use far-flung donors; the donated milk is flown on ice to the milk bank.)

And don't forget the grapevine: Other nursing moms often are excellent resources for recommending good lactation consultants. If you don't know any, call the local La Leche League, or a store that specializes in maternity and baby products.

A good lactation consultant will observe you with the baby to check out his latch-on and positioning, and will watch how he nurses—all things that are impossible to do over the phone. A good lactation consultant will also listen to you without constantly interrupting or finishing your sentences (two clues that she's not really listening to what you're saying.) When you're searching for a lactation consultant, let people know what sort of personality you'd like best—relaxed, formal, technical, casual—to help narrow down the candidates.

By the way, you'd be doing the hospital a favor if you let the OB department director know about your experience with the staff lactation consultant. It's possible you caught her on a bad day, but if she's habitually abrupt with new moms, her supervisors should be aware of that. And if she's not a certified member of the International Lactation Consultants Association (ILCA), complain. ILCA members go through a lengthy accreditation process, and they keep up in continuing education programs.

See also La Leche League; Milk Banks; Appendix

Lactose Intolerance

Q: My newborn won't latch on right most of the time. When he does, both he and I are in pain. A nurse at the hospital said that he might be lactose intolerant—that he's allergic to my milk. Is that possible?

A: If your baby is truly lactose intolerant, you wouldn't be able to breastfeed him. Breast milk has twice as much lactose as cow's milk. However, lactose intolerance is extremely rare in infants.

It's more likely that your son isn't latching on correctly, which is why your nipples hurt and he's upset—he can't get enough milk.

It's possible that he is sensitive to something in your diet. Intolerance of dairy, soy, and wheat products results in gas, cramps, diarrhea, bloating, incessant fussiness, or yeast infections similar to those seen in adults who are lactose intolerant. (A dairy sensitivity would help explain why your nipples are so sore: One symptom is thrush, which makes your nipples exquisitely sensitive. Thrush is unusual with a newborn, but it can happen.)

The nurse who advised you may be relying on outdated information. If your doctor feels that she's correct, it's possible to test for true lactose intolerance, which is a genetic disorder.

Odds are that something else is causing the problem. See an IBCLC lactation consultant to help resolve your difficulties and to demonstrate nursing techniques.

See also Allergies, Dairy; Allergies (Baby's), About; Lactation Consultant; Latching On, About; Thrush, About

Large Breasts

Q: My breasts are size 44EE. Most of the nursing techniques that my smaller friends use don't work for me. Do you have any tips for extra-large-sized breastfeeding?

A: The basics are the same: a good latch, adequate back and arm support, and correct positioning. But you're right: breastfeeding is different for well-endowed moms.

1. *Invest in a good nursing bra.* You need to support your breast, as well as the baby, when you nurse and when you're not nursing. If you have large breasts, a good nursing bra is essential. Go to a store that has a fitting expert to make sure you find a bra that is best for you.

Off-the-rack (or off-the-Internet) nursing bras (including Goddess 510, Leading Lady, and Motherwear Extra Support) are available in sizes up to a 48J. Several companies design custom-made bras. Bra back extenders are helpful in late pregnancy and during the early days of engorgement, when your size increases temporarily. (The extenders are removable when your body settles into its post-birth size.) If you can't find a bra locally that fits you, go to breastfeeding Web sites online and look for links to sources that sell nursing bras.

Never wear a bra that is persistently uncomfortable. A good nursing bra unfastens easily in front, supports your breast without pressing against your breast tissue, washes well, and fits you comfortably. Wash your nursing bra with a weak solution of bleach and hot water several times a week. Most moms have at least two nursing bras—one to wear while the other is being laundered.

Avoid underwire bras; the wires press against breast tissue and are notorious for causing plugged ducts. If a bra is too loose, it will ride up or down, causing sore breasts, plugged ducts, and uneven drainage problems.

Bras that are too tight can inhibit your milk supply and can also cause plugged ducts.

2. Keep your breasts clean. Women with large breasts are prone to skin infections and irritations under their breasts. Topical yeast infections (in the folds of your skin) are common in pregnancy and can mean that you're more susceptible to thrush.

Wash your breasts daily with water. Don't use soap, body gel, shampoo, or scent on your nipples; these things can dry and irritate your skin. After you wash, use a towel to dry thoroughly, and pay special attention to the skin under your breasts. Use a portable blow-drier to make sure that your skin is completely dry. Even a little moisture causes or worsens a yeast infection. Never put talcum or cornstarch under your breasts—they only feed yeast infections.

3. Let the baby nurse frequently, and on demand. Forget the advice to limit a baby to 5 to 10 minutes per breast. Newborns frequently need 10 to 20 minutes per breast, and slow or sleepy nursers may need up to 40 minutes per breast. It's okay to nurse on just one breast at a feed, as long as you offer the other breast for the next session. Babies generally need to nurse 8 to 12 times in 24 hours. If your baby doesn't wake at least every 3 hours, tickle him, rub his back, or pat his bare foot with a damp, cool washcloth.

4. Massage your breasts while breastfeeding. Gently stroking your breasts while nursing makes sure that the milk sinuses all empty, and will help avoid plugged ducts and other problems.

5. Have patience. It usually takes a baby a lot of time—latching over and over—before she learns to open her mouth wide enough to latch on and get the hang of breastfeeding. There's a learning curve for you, too—figuring out how to smoosh your nipple into a sandwich that fits into the baby's mouth, finding the most comfortable nursing positions, etc. There will be days when you feel like you've done nothing but nurse, or try to nurse, over and over. (Consider this good training for the toddler years, when your child clamors for the same book and video dozens of times a day.)

TROUBLESHOOTING

Chronic thrush and/or other topical yeast infections: Get a new set of nursing bras if you can afford it. If not, soak the bras in a vinegar rinse (half water and half vinegar), and hang to dry in the sun.

Nursing in public: Use the cradle hold, and cover up with a blanket. Wear two-piece outfits (loose-fitting top over shorts or pants) to make nursing easier and more discreet. If you're self-conscious, practice nursing in front of a mirror, or nursing in a supportive group—with other moms you know, or at a La Leche League group meeting.

Small baby and big breasts: The football hold is best when your breast weighs more than your baby. Nurse frequently and on demand. If your breasts are too engorged for the baby to latch onto, express some milk before trying to latch him on. If your baby is a preemie or extremely small, you may need to pump until she can nurse. Avoid nipple confusion by feeding the baby with an eyedropper or syringe if you'll only be pumping for a few days; or use a sippy cup, spoon, paladai, or tube feeding system if it's a week or more before she'll be able to breastfeed.

See also Nursing Bras, About; Paladai; Positions, About; Tube Feeding Lactation Aid; Thrush, About

Laser Vision Correcting Surgery

See Vision Correcting Surgery and Breastfeeding

Latching On, About

Does breastfeeding hurt? A proper latch-on is the key to eliminating pain during the early weeks post partum. In most cases, painful nursing is reduced or eliminated by getting your baby correctly on the breast and finding the right position.

Start by sitting comfortably. You may need pillows behind your back for support and a stool to support your feet. Elevating your feet brings up your lap and knees, making it easier to hold the baby. You can buy a breastfeeding stool, but any small footrest will do the job.

Before starting to nurse, put your finger in your baby's mouth and feel for the place where the hard palate meets the soft palate—it's quite far back in her mouth. That's how deep she'll need to pull in your nipple when she nurses, which is why it's so important to give her a big mouthful of areola as well as your nipple.

Sit all the way back in your chair. Bring the baby to you, instead of leaning down to the baby. (That strains your back, and makes it more difficult to correctly latch on and position the baby.)

Use one hand to support the business end of your breast. The best support position is the C-hold, with the thumb of your hand on top of your breast, and the rest of your fingers underneath. (Make sure your fingers do not touch the areola.) A common mistake: the "cigarette hold"—holding your nipple instead of the breast, which makes it impossible for your baby to get a good mouthful of areola, pinches your nipple, and facilitates cracked, painful nipples.

Hold your baby close as you nurse; the baby's nose should just touch your breast. (Don't worry; she has enough room to breathe. A baby's nose is wide, with flared nostrils to accommodate nursing.) If she seems to have trouble breathing—gasping and unlatching—lower the elbow of your cradling arm just a bit. (Don't drop your elbow, or your baby will unlatch.)

Make sure the baby's upper ear, shoulder, and hip are in a straight line. She shouldn't have to twist her neck to get at your breast.

Be persistent. It takes time for a mom and a baby to get used to each other. It can take 2 or 3 weeks, sometimes longer, for a

baby to breastfeed easily. By the time your baby is 6 weeks old, breastfeeding should be second nature for both of you.
See also Latching On, Refusal

Latching On Correctly

Q: I dread breastfeeding time. When my 2-week-old son latches on, it feels as if a C-clamp is crunching my nipple. How can I tell if he's latched on correctly?

A: First, make sure you're giving him a big mouthful of nipple AND areola. Wait until he's opening his mouth as wide as he can, as if he's yawning. If he's not opening widely enough, point your nipple at the roof of his mouth, and slide it from one end of his lips to the other—like pulling a zipper. (You can also pull his mouth along your nipple, in the same motion.) Wait for him to open wide before bringing him to your breast.

If his mouth isn't wide open, he won't be able to empty your milk ducts.

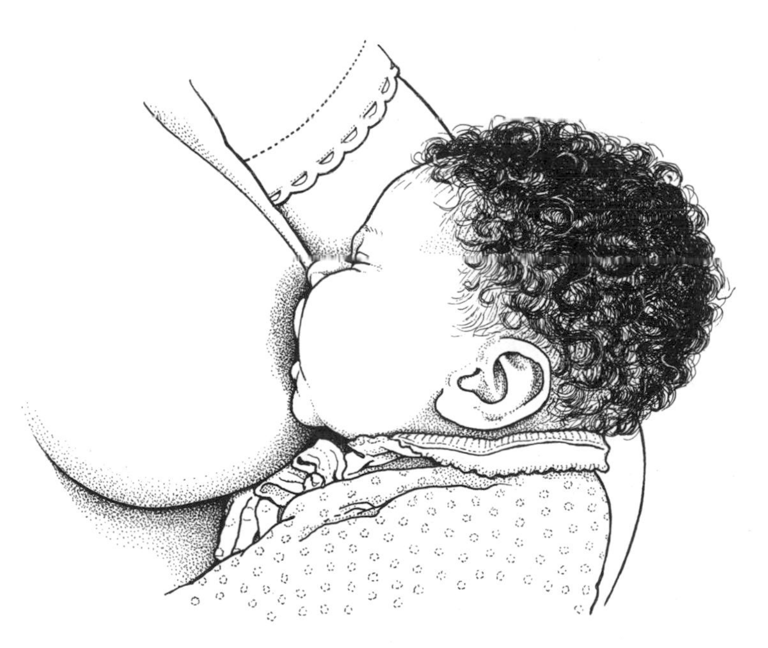

When his chin touches your breast, pull him close against your breast, pointing your nipple at the back of his mouth, and get as much areola as possible in his mouth. (If he's latching on only to your nipple, all that pain is for nothing—he's not getting as much milk as he needs.)

You can check his latch by pulling down his lower lip. You should be able to see his tongue. If you can't see his tongue, use one finger to gently pull down on his chin, so his lower lip pokes out in an exaggerated half-pout.

See also Breast Compression; Lactation Consultant

Latching On, Refusal

Q: It took 6 days for my milk to come in, and I was recovering from a cesarean. My daughter isn't keen on nursing. I've been pumping and feeding her expressed milk, supplemented with formula. She drinks well from the bottle, but I wish she'd breastfeed. After 2 weeks, is it time to give up on breastfeeding?

A: No, it's not too late. You'll need patience and persistence—your daughter may have nipple confusion, and she's learned that it's easier to drink from a bottle than to nurse. If she had a suction tube in her throat to remove excess mucus after birth, her throat may be sore.

Get some help from a lactation consultant. Once you establish breastfeeding, you may need another visit from the midwife or lactation consultant for some fine-tuning.

When she's ready to nurse, position her so she's facing your nipple. Pull her close, aiming your nipple at the back of her mouth. Her chin should be pushing into your breast under your nipple, and her nose up and away from the breast above your nipple. Her lips should be flanged—slightly turned out. Carefully pull down her lower lip: You should be able to see her tongue between her lips and your nipple.

Don't worry about whether she can breathe. If she's properly latched on and positioned, she'll be fine. A baby who can't breathe will pull off the breast.

Important: Get good, reliable help. A lactation consultant, midwife, or La Lache League leader can work one-to-one with you. Find someone you like, and work with her.

One trick: Just before nursing, put warm, damp washcloths on your nipples. This helps stimulate letdown. Then, when you're latching her on, make a "nipple sandwich"—press on both sides of the aureola and pop the works into her mouth when she opens wide. If milk jets out, wait until the flow slows down before trying to latch her on.

See also Breast Compression; Lactation Consultants; Nipple Confusion; Overactive Letdown; Positions, About

Latching On, Clamping Down

Q: My 2-day-old daughter clamps on like a vise. Is there anything I can do to lessen the awesome power of this reflex? If this is what breastfeeding is like, no wonder so many moms give up!

A: Many newborns tend to clamp down pretty hard for the first week or two. Eventually, they learn to relax when they latch on. Until then, you can help her relax by supporting her jaw as she nurses. Place your hand, palm up, under your breast, with your index finger and thumb on each side of her jaw. Avoid grasping her jaw. Just support it. This is tricky at first. Get a lactation consultant to help you with this. She should watch you practice until this feels natural.

Another suggestion: Lie down with the baby in bed, naked from the waist up, with the baby in only a diaper. Lie on your back, and put her on your stomach between your breasts. As she roots to seek out your nipple, guide her mouth and help her nurse in this tummy-to-tummy position. This often helps a baby's jaw relax enough to feel more comfortable.

Hang in there! Usually this problem resolves itself within 10 days.

See also Positions, About

Latching On and Off

Q: When she latches on, my 2-day-old daughter nurses like a champ. But she'll just get latched on, and then pops off again and fusses, and we have to start all over. It's very frustrating. She latches on well enough to stimulate my letdown reflex, so milk sprays out. Both of us get drenched. How can I get her to stay latched on?

A: Sounds as if you have an overactive letdown. That's usually why newborns and infants pop on and off the breast. The milk flows so fast and so strong that they can't swallow fast enough to keep up, so they stop nursing to breathe.

Try expressing a little milk before you start feeding her. Hand-express some milk for 30 seconds or so, until the milk stops spraying so forcefully. And keep plenty of clean towels or cloth diapers around! If she continues to latch on and off, even after you've expressed some milk and tried other techniques to mitigate overactive letdown, ask a lactation consultant for help. Is she latching on properly? Could she be allergic to something in your diet?

See also Allergies (Baby's), About; Distracted Baby; Latching On, About; Overactive Letdown; Thrush, About

Leaking, About

If you're a mother with an overactive or strong letdown, stock up on nursing pads, and zip your silk blouses into a garment bag until you're well past the weaning stage. Women who have a vigorous milk supply may still be able to express milk months (and even years) after their child has weaned. They don't need to wear nursing pads forever, but they may find themselves with a spontaneous damp spot or two on the bra at unexpected moments. Hearing a baby cry—even on TV or radio—or having an orgasm, or sometimes even just thinking about nursing can trigger your breasts to produce a drop of milk. This isn't a big deal. (Exception: If one or both of your nipples produces a daily discharge, and you're not pregnant or breastfeeding, it may be a sign of cancer. See your physician immediately.)

While you're breastfeeding, expect to use nursing pads daily for the first 3 months, and longer if you have a vigorous letdown. When you're nursing your baby on one breast, it's not unusual if the other breast starts to let down, too. If you're deft, and you need to stockpile milk, you can pump the other breast as the baby's nursing—many moms swear this method collects the most milk. Or you can press a cloth diaper or a burp cloth over the leaking nipple to discourage the letdown.

Your breasts may leak at night, especially if they are engorged. (This is the downside of having a baby who sleeps for long stretches at night!) If your breasts are so engorged that you can't sleep, you can get up and pump. Otherwise, sleep on top of a thick towel, or keep a towel near the bed so you can arrange it under your chest if you feel yourself starting to leak.

During the day, nursing pads help. Change them as soon as they feel wet. (Damp nursing pads stiffen when they dry, irritating your nipples. They can also lead to bacterial growth and breast infections.) If you leak heavily, especially if you wake up soaked at night, try folding a washcloth or a cloth diaper cut in half in each bra cup.

Cabbage leaves can help control leaking by relieving engorgement. Don't use them if you're having milk supply problems—cabbage leaves are a longstanding aid for weaning mothers—but they can be a godsend if you're frustrated by an overactive letdown.

See also Cabbage Leaves; Overactive Letdown; Weaning, About

Leaking After Weaning

Q: My breast started leaking milk during foreplay last night, even though I weaned my last child 3 years ago. I think it's sympathetic lactating—my sister's pregnant with twins. Could it be?

A: Probably not. You should see your doctor if you continue to produce milk. Although some mothers can continue to express milk long after weaning, spontaneous leaking is less common. What you experienced may be related to medications you're taking, or to abnormal levels of prolactin, a pituitary tumor, or other situations that require medical attention.

Leaking at Night

Q: The good news: My baby's sleeping through the night! (Well, for 6 hours at a stretch.) The bad news: My breasts leak so much at night that the sheets get soaked. Waterproof mattress pads are too uncomfortable, and they just make me sweat more. I don't wear a night bra because I was getting plugged ducts and infections. What should I do?

A: Try sleeping on a large cotton towel (use a hand towel when you sleep on your back; tuck it under your torso to keep it in place) or a cotton crib pad. Some nursing mothers keep a stack of cloth diapers (the thick, prefolded kind) by the bedside, replacing damp diapers with dry ones.

Some women wear a sports bra instead of a traditional nursing bra at night. Because they're mostly Lycra, sports bras are stretchy. They'll hold nursing pads in place without compressing the breast tissue as some nursing bras do. Sports bras don't offer much support, but they're fine if all you need is something to prevent chafing and to hold nursing pads in place.

Letdown, Identifying

Q: I have no clue what other moms are talking about when they say their milk lets down. I don't feel a thing when I nurse my baby (6 days old). Should I be feeling something?

A: Not necessarily. Some women don't feel the letdown sensation. Others feel their nipples tingle—sometimes the tingling feels almost like static electricity—and their breasts swell perceptibly a few seconds before and during letdown. Every woman reacts differently.

Letdown, Painful

Q: After some problems, I've finally established a nursing relationship with my 5-week-old daughter. But I still feel some pain during letdown. It's sort of an electric feeling. What can I do about it?

A: Unfortunately, letdown is uncomfortable or even painful for some women—a sensation somewhere between being pinched and feeling a mild electrical shock. It's often worse when you're engorged and the milk-producing cells higher in the breast tissue force the milk down into the ducts. It should get less painful in time. Meanwhile, you can take a breastfeeding-friendly pain reliever, like Tylenol, to numb things a bit.

If the unused breast simultaneously lets down, use a soft cloth diaper or towel—or a bottle, if your coordination is good—to catch the excess. (It can be up to an ounce or so, enough to save and freeze for a future feeding.) Do not try to block the leak by pressing against it—that can lead to plugged ducts and worse.

If the pain during letdown is new, it may be an early sign of thrush.

See also Thrush, About

Letdown, Stimulating

Q: I'm a brand-new mom, and it's a struggle to get a letdown for my week-old baby. I've tried massage, but it doesn't seem to help much. The baby and I are both frustrated. What can I do to get my letdown going?

A: Your milk is still coming in, so keep trying to nurse. The baby's nursing will help stimulate the flow. Are you drinking enough water and other fluids? (Hint: If your urine is yellow, you're not drinking enough.) You should be drinking at least 8 to 10 ounces of water an hour.

One short-term fix for your problem is oxytocin nasal spray. It's available only by prescription, and you'll need to talk to your obstetrician about why you want it and how to use it. If your doctor is agreeable, the spray will prompt a letdown. However, you can use the spray only for a few days—less than a week, max—but it may help jump-start your breastfeeding relationship enough to give both you and your baby confidence.

See also Breast Compression; Relaxing While Nursing

Lidocaine

See Dental Work and Breastfeeding

Lipase, Excess

Q: I've just started pumping milk for my son. He refuses to take even a drop. My husband thought the milk smelled funny, even though I'd just pumped it. He tasted it and said it tasted like vomit. I didn't believe him till I tried it, too. The expressed milk in the freezer is the same way. What am I doing wrong?

A: You're in the company of women who have excess lipase in their milk—a dubious distinction that means extra work if you're planning on pumping.

Lipase is an enzyme that helps break down fat, and its enzymatic activity increases when it gets cold. In other words, excess lipase basically partially digests the milk.

This isn't a problem when the baby is nursing, because when he's suckling, the breast milk's temperature is warm and constant. But expressing the milk nudges the extra lipase into action, wasting your pumping efforts if you store the milk without treating it.

The easiest (we use the word guardedly) solution is to scald the milk after expressing it. Normally, breast milk should not be heated or boiled, but if you want to give your baby only breast milk, you don't have much choice. Heated breast milk loses some of its benefits—some antibacterial qualities in particular—though the loss is minimal. (Human milk banks also heat the milk donated to them, but nutritionists still consider the boiled milk superior to formula.) So, it's up to you to decide whether it's worth the extra effort.

See also Sour/Spoiled Breast Milk

Long Nipples

See Nipples, Long

Lopsided Nursing

Q: My 2-month-old nurses more often on my right breast than the left. It leaves me lopsided. My aunt told me to put honey on the left nipple to get her to nurse more equally. Would that help?

A: No, but it might give your baby a case of botulism. Honey is a no-no for babies and children under age 2. You can try latching her onto the right breast, and then switching her to the left side in mid-feed. Or, if it doesn't bother you, don't worry about it. Some women nurse only from one breast—either because the baby has a breast preference, or there's a problem with the other breast.

See also Prefers One Breast

Lump, Breast

See Breast Lump

Lump in Armpit

Q: I have a painful lump just under the crease of my arm. It feels like a plugged duct, but it's too far from my breast to be a milk duct. What is it?

A: It's probably a plugged duct, even though it's closer to your armpit than your nipple. A plugged duct can occur in any part of your breast tissue, including the tissue under your arm. The best way to treat a plugged duct is to continue nursing frequently on the affected breast and to wear loose clothing and bras without underwires. Applying heat will help, too.

See your doctor to rule out other possibilities.

See also Breast Lump; Plugged Ducts, About

M

Marijuana

Q: Before I was pregnant, I smoked marijuana now and then. Now that my son's born, I think about smoking again. Can marijuana chemicals get in your breast milk? How long will it stay there?

A: The American Academy of Pediatrics' Committee on Drugs states that marijuana is contraindicated for use by breastfeeding mothers. (Marijuana is also an illegal substance in the United States.) Research indicates that the tetrahydrocannabinol (THC) in marijuana rapidly enters your bloodstream. Levels of THC peak in breast milk within an hour of your inhaling marijuana smoke. Residual THC in breast milk is potent enough to affect a baby's own blood chemistry for up to 1 month; the THC shows up in a baby's urine 2 to 3 weeks after the mother has smoked marijuana. Exposure to THC increases a baby's risk for sudden infant death syndrome and for decreased motor development, and it may alter her brain cells.

Mastitis, About

One doctor described mastitis as "a bunch of germs having a party in your milk ducts"—a wry description of an otherwise humorless affliction. Mastitis is a vicious infection that develops fast and, untreated, can quickly get worse. This is one party you don't want to throw.

The germs that cause mastitis can enter through the nipple when the baby falls asleep while nursing: The pores in your nipple are still open, giving the germs easy access. Other causes include a too-tight nursing bra or sleep bra, bunching your clothes under your arms while you nurse (that puts pressure on the milk ducts), opening your nursing bra flap just enough to let the baby get at your nipple (allowing the pressure of the flap to cause problems not only with plugged ducts and mastitis, but also with nursing), or frequently missing a regular nursing session.

Mastitis usually begins with symptoms like a sore, painful breast, accompanied by feeling punchy and feverish. Sometimes you'll find a small lump, warm to the touch, near your nipple. If you use a breast pump, you may notice that the milk from the affected breast is unusually thick, almost like cream soup; in rare cases, clots or clumps form in the collection bottle.

If you catch the symptoms early, you can stop them from developing into full-blown mastitis by applying warm compresses, massaging the lump (toward your nipple), resting in bed, and nursing and pumping as much as possible on the affected breast. You won't want to—it'll hurt—but mastitis hurts more.

Occasionally, mastitis shows up with no warning, like a party-crasher. You may feel as if you're getting a bad case of the flu—shivery, sweaty, with a terrific headache. Once you develop a fever and/or chills, you're dealing with mastitis, not a plugged duct. The solution is prescription antibiotics. The drugs take effect swiftly. You'll feel better within hours, and the infection will be resolved within 48 hours—but keep taking the drugs for the prescribed period, and try to get as much bed rest as possible for at least a couple of days after your symptoms are gone. Mastitis often recurs in moms who skip bed rest and resume their regular (overloaded) schedule too soon.

If the infection fails to respond to the antibiotics, go back to your doctor immediately. You may need a different antibiotic. Several antibiotics are used to treat mastitis and other bacterial infections; Keflex, Dicloxycillin, Augmentin, and Cipro are widely used. If a second course of antibiotics doesn't work, ask your doctor to do a culture and reassess the situation.

When you're taking an antibiotic, add acidophilus to your diet (in the form of supplements or yogurt with an active culture, not frozen yogurt) to help stave off yeast infections, which can provoke more plugged ducts. Ibuprofen will help reduce swelling and fever.

To relieve the pain, fill a cotton sock with dry (uncooked) white rice. Put it in the microwave oven for 1 minute. It will be hot when you remove it, but also moist—an ideal warm compress. Apply it to the affected part of your breast for at least 1 minute, preferably longer, before you nurse. (If it's too hot, use a thin cotton blanket or washcloth as a buffer.) The heat will help dilate your milk ducts and help empty the plugged duct(s).

Continue breastfeeding while you're under treatment. The more often you nurse, the more quickly you'll clear any plugged ducts. Try varying the nursing position to make sure all the ducts are fully drained. It may (probably will) hurt, especially at first, but this is the best way to deal with mastitis.

Untreated, mastitis can get much worse. It can develop into a breast abscess—a nasty situation that's more complicated to treat, often requiring minor surgery—and you'll end up on antibiotics anyway. For the baby's sake and your own, nip mastitis in the bud as soon as you recognize the symptoms.

If you're squeamish about prescription drugs, you can try treating mastitis with colloidal silver, a natural substance composed of submicroscopic clusters of silver suspended in ionized water. Colloidal silver is a powerful and nontoxic antibiotic that is increasingly popular as an alternative medicine. The University of California/Los Angeles medical labs found that it killed every virus they tested.

However, even though the manufacturers of colloidal silver say that it's safe for pregnant and lactating women, use it prudently. A 1996 medical research report assessing the risks and benefits of colloidal silver found that indiscriminate use can lead to toxicity. Colloidal silver is sold through whole food and health food stores.

Should the mastitis persist (or return) after you've finished your course of antibiotics, ask your doctor to culture your milk so the lab can determine what kind of bacteria is causing your problem.

See also Clumping Milk; Plugged Ducts, About; Pumping, About

Mastitis and Nursing

Q: I'm on antibiotics because I have mastitis in my right breast. It is still extremely hard, tender, and sore. My baby won't nurse on that side because my nipple is so taut that he can't latch on properly. My doctor wants me to nurse the affected breast. Can't I just pump that breast, and nurse him on the other side?

A: Sorry, but your doctor is right. It's extremely important to continue nursing your baby on the affected breast when you have mastitis. You must get the engorgement down immediately. Once the breast is less engorged, your nipple will be more pliant and less painful. Every hour and a half to 2 hours, empty your breast—preferably by nursing, but by hand or with a pump if the baby absolutely refuses to nurse on that side. (Caveat: If your nipple is excruciatingly tight, a pump will hurt less and work faster than trying to nurse.) Emptying that breast frequently and fully will help you heal faster. It also keeps up your milk supply.

Before attempting to nurse or express milk, use a warm, moist compress or a saline soak. Fill a large measuring cup or basin with warm water, add a teaspoon of salt for every cup for water, and immerse the breast by leaning forward over the water for about 10 minutes.

When you're severely engorged—when your breast feels like an unhappily overripe cantaloupe—express for no longer than 10 minutes at a time. If you can tolerate using a pump, put it on the lowest (intermittent) pressure setting to reduce the risk of damaging your delicate breast tissue. (You may need to hand-express once or twice before you're comfortable enough to use a pump, and you'll still probably need to hand-express a little bit of milk before putting on the pump cups.)

If you have severe pain, use an ice pack (a cold pack or a package of frozen peas) on the affected breast for about 15 minutes between feeding (or expressing) sessions. The cold will help reduce the pain and swelling, just as heat stimulates letdown. If you need more pain relief, the American Academy of Pediatrics considers ibuprofen compatible with breastfeeding.

He may not want to nurse on that side, not only because

you're so engorged but also because when mastitis is present, your milk tastes salty (only in the affected breast). Babies prefer sweet milk to salty milk. If he refuses to nurse on the infected breast, pump until it's empty. You may need to pump again at the next feeding session (try to get him to nurse first), but after a couple of pumping sessions, the milk in that breast should taste sweet again.
See also Mastitis, About; Plugged Ducts, About

Meclizine

Q: I'm susceptible to motion sickness, and previously I've controlled that with meclizine. I'm breastfeeding a 3-month-old, and about to go on a 3-day car trip. Does meclizine leach into breast milk? My doctor doesn't know.
A: No data are available on meclizine's transfer to human milk, but it has been studied in dogs. The levels in dog milk are low: Only 3 percent of the dose transferred to milk. Meclizine is effective for vertigo, nausea and vomiting, and motion sickness, and until recently it was routinely used by pregnant women to treat morning sickness. The main contraindication for meclizine, as with other antihistamines, is that it's a sedative and conceivably can increase the risk of sudden infant death because of its sedating effect, so bear that in mind during your trip. An alternative anti-nausea treatment is ginger. Chewing on raw ginger, candied ginger, or the pickled slices used as a sushi condiment may mitigate your motion illness.
See also Allergies (Yours), About

Medications and Breast Milk

Q: I had to quit nursing my first child because I was worried that different medicines I had to take for colds, allergies and other problems would be passed on through the milk and might harm her. Can you help? I'm expecting our second child in 2 months, and I'd like to nurse again, but she arrives in the middle of cold and flu season.

A: Actually, there are few medications that breastfeeding moms cannot have. However, there are several things to consider when you take medications (over-the-counter, prescription, or herbal remedies). Some, like antihistamines or birth control pills containing estrogen, can cause your milk supply to decrease. And how your body absorbs medication—over-the-counter, prescription, or herbal supplements—can vary, sometimes dramatically, from one person to another. If you're concerned about how a medication will affect your breast milk, or if you're worried about how medications, including herbal supplements and vitamins, might interact, you should consult your doctor or a pharmacist.

Most medications do leach into breast milk. The amounts vary from a trace to such significant levels that the medication should be avoided. Medications that routinely are prescribed for babies—amoxicillin, for example—are not a concern. If a certain medication is not recommended for a nursing mother, there usually are alternatives. (Zoloft, for example, is a breastfeeding-friendly alternative to the antidepressant Prozac.)

When you take a medication, over-the-counter or prescription, time your doses so the baby gets the lowest amount possible in your milk. (To determine this, find out how long the drug's half-life is and how quickly it is metabolized.) The best way to minimize the chance of passing on any drugs through your milk is to nurse just before you take the medication.

Some drugs have side effects that present a danger to a nursing baby. Even if only a small amount of those drugs were to pass into your milk, the medication would not be compatible with breastfeeding. If you're concerned about whether a drug presents problems to a nursing baby, the definitive reference book is Thomas Hale's *Medications and Mother's Milk* ($22.95, plus shipping costs; to order, call 800-378-1317).

There also is a lactation hot line that provides accurate, current information on medication and breast milk. Call 806-358-8138 for information about signing up for the hot line. If you have a fax machine, call 806-356-9556 and enter 1 as your password; the system will fax a registration form and information.

See also Allergies (Baby's), About

Menstruation, Resuming, About

Once you've finished your postpartum mega-period—that 2-week marathon, with a few days of heavy bleeding followed by lighter bleeding and spotting for 10 days or so—it can be months before you resume your normal menstrual cycle, particularly if you breastfeed exclusively. This doesn't mean you can't get pregnant. You can get pregnant while you're breastfeeding, even if you haven't had a period yet. And, as the most basic sex-ed handbooks will tell you, it's possible to get pregnant if you've had only one period.

Technically, it's possible to get pregnant even before your period resumes if you ovulate before the first period.

Some women, including those who breastfeed exclusively, find that their period returns a couple of months after their baby's birth. Some women don't resume their periods until a month or so after they've weaned the baby. Many women find, to their exasperation, that their periods resume within the first 6 months to a year of the baby's birth but that their cycles are erratic as long as they continue breastfeeding. In other words, this is strictly a Your Mileage May Vary situation. The main rule: Assume you're fertile until proved otherwise.

However, if you resume bleeding within the first 6 weeks of the baby's birth, the blood may be lochia. If you've been bleeding consistantly since the baby's birth, with only a brief interval or two of not bleeding during that 6-week span, you should see your OB/GYN. Retained placental material is bad news and needs immediate medical attention.

Many women find that their milk supply is lower just before and during their menstrual periods. The dip is only temporary, and babies respond by nursing more frequently. You can help keep up your supply by eating a little more protein before and during your menstrual period and by taking calcium and magnesium supplements—but if you take other medications, especially to treat blood pressure, ask your physician before taking supplements.

Many mothers find that their breasts and nipples are exceptionally sensitive when they ovulate and/or menstruate. Sometimes that sensitivity crosses the threshold into the sort of pain that accompanies thrush. There's not much you can do about this, although warm compresses may offer some relief.

If your period fails to resume within 3 months after you wean the baby, or after you've cut back dramatically on nursing sessions (supplementing with formula, feeding more solids, etc.), you should consult your OB/GYN. Some women need hormone therapy to jump-start their periods again. Even though it's nice to avoid the monthly hassle, consistently missing your period may be a warning sign of other trouble.

Menstruating Already?

Q: I've been breastfeeding, exclusively and on demand, my 2-month-old daughter. Imagine my surprise when, 6 weeks after she was delivered, I got my period again! I'm exasperated. One of the advantages of breastfeeding, I thought, was an extended vacation from menstruating. Is this common?

A: Occasionally, but not often, a nursing mom does begin menstruating again within a couple of months after her baby's birth. It's possible that what you experienced was a pseudoperiod—a single bleeding episode that sometimes occurs 5 to 7 weeks after birth—and that you won't truly begin menstruating again for months.

Microwave Heating Expressed Milk

Q: We always microwave cow's milk to heat it for our children, but our pediatrician told us not to thaw frozen breast milk in the microwave. Why not?

A: Pediatricians advise against heating breast milk in the

microwave because the milk heats unevenly. Hot spots can burn a baby's mouth and esophagus. Microwave-heated milk—human and cow milk—has burned some babies' mouths so severely that they were admitted to hospitals for treatment.
See also Pumping, About

Milk in Baby's Nipples

See Witches' Milk

Milk, Donating

Q: My DD cups literally floweth over: I can pump about 240 cubic centimeters (8 ounces) at one session. So far I've filled my freezer, and part of the freezer at work, with expressed milk. There's no more storage space, and I still have to pump. I don't want to throw out the extra milk, and I know there are babies who need it. How can I find those families?

A: Get in touch with a human milk bank. There are less than a dozen milk banks in North America, and usually they desperately need milk from qualified donors, especially from mothers of preterm babies.

Milk banks are quite strict and require blood tests as well as exacting high hygienic standards from qualified donors. Qualifications include fully lactating women in excellent health, nonsmoking, with thriving babies and no history of hepatitis, illicit IV drug use, or intimate contact with anyone at risk for HIV or AIDS. The extensive screening process requires a blood test against communicable diseases, including hepatitis B, hepatitis C, HIV (AIDS), HTLV-I, and HTLV-II.

However, if you pass the screening process, milk banks may be able to accept milk pumped before you are evaluated as a donor, particularly if you pumped milk for a premature infant.

Milk banks are nonprofit organizations. However, their milk must be purchased, and it is available only by a doctor's prescription. Financial aid is available for families who need it.

Babies who need donor milk to survive are rarely turned away for lack of money. Some insurance companies will reimburse part or all of the expenses related to donor milk.

Some resources:

- Human Milk Banking Association, 8 Jan Sebastian Way #13, Sandwich, MA 02563; 888-232-8809
- HealthOne Mother's Milk Bank, 1719 E. 19th Ave., Denver, CO 80218; 303-869-1888
- Mother's Milk Bank, Valley Medical Center, P.O. Box 5730, San Jose, CA 95150; 408-998-4550

Milk, Green

See Green Breast Milk

Milk in Mother's Diet

See Calcium in Mother's Diet; Nonfat Milk for Nursing Mothers

Milk Banks, Receiving Milk from

Q: I've heard about milk banks that collect human breast milk. How can I get in touch with one of them? I have a low supply—I can only get an ounce or two when I pump—and I'd prefer to supplement with breast milk rather than with formula.

A: There are only a handful of milk banks in North America, and they're a far cry from being the equivalent of a 7-Eleven for mother's milk. A milk bank's milk is earmarked for babies whose health is seriously impaired—an inability to digest formula, failure-to-thrive problems, or a birth mother at risk for immune deficiency illnesses, for example.

Many people are surprised that the milk is available only by prescription. And it's not free: The going rate is $2.50 per ounce, which pays for processing and transporting donor milk. Some insurance companies cover part or all of the cost.

Talk to your pediatrician. If she feels that your baby has a med-

ical need for donor milk, she can help make arrangements.
See also Milk, Donating; Appendix

Milk Blisters

Q: I'm worried about the persistent presence of white dots on my nipples. They won't go away, and they hurt. I scratched one, and it had pus inside, like a pimple. It's not thrush: the baby has no symptoms. My 3-month-old just started teething, and nursing is so painful that I'm having trouble coping.

A: If it's not thrush, then it could be milk blisters. (If there is only one white dot, it's known as a bleb and usually accompanies a plugged duct. Several blebs indicate thrush.) Usually, they appear on the upper areola and can take from a few days to heal. Milk blisters typically are caused by plugs of thick milk that seal over and get inflamed. (Comparing milk blisters to pimples is unappetizing but apt.)

Treat milk blisters as you would plugged ducts. Before you nurse, put warm compresses on your nipples to soften the blisters. Then nurse as often as possible. (If the baby won't nurse that often, use a breast pump.) With luck and persistence, your baby will suckle off the plugs (with no harm to the baby). Between feeds, use ice packs to numb the pain, chilling your nipples for 15 or 20 minutes at a stretch.

If the blisters fail to clear up, you may be dealing with thrush, even if your baby seems to have no symptoms. Thrush is definitely a possibility if your nipples start to burn or get tender and itchy, or if you start to feel electric pains shooting from your nipple to your chest.

Even if it's not thrush, ask your OB/GYN to look at the blisters. Some milk blisters need to be evacuated with office surgery.
See also Bleb; Plugged Ducts, About; Thrush, About

Milk: Low Supply

Q: I worry that I don't have enough milk for my newborn son. When I pump, I barely get an ounce. After 4 days of trying to breastfeed him, we started supplementing with a syringe next to my nipple. That screwed up his latch-on, and we began using Avent bottles to feed him expressed milk. He's 2 weeks old now, and I'm still not making enough milk—he's only barely regained his birth weight. The nurse at my pediatrician's office told me I might as well switch to formula, since my supply is so low. What can I do?

A: Most babies regain their birth weight within the first week, but some babies take longer. Once the baby regains his birth weight, he should be gaining about half a pound a week. Your situation is more indicative of feeding difficulties, which can be fixed, than milk supply problems. In other words, your baby isn't nursing properly—he's not able to get the milk your breasts do produce, which means your breasts make less and less milk in response.

Pumping is not an accurate measurement of your milk supply—it reflects how much you can pump, not how much you can produce. (However, regular pumping can help increase your milk supply.)

Are you drinking enough? Is your urine very light yellow or clear? Are you resting, even a little? Is your baby producing 8 to 12 wet and poopy diapers in 24 hours? If the answers are yes, then you're making enough milk. But if your baby isn't producing stools, he is not getting enough to eat. Very few wet diapers indicates dangerous dehydration.

If your baby is losing weight, and failing to produce even eight wet or soiled diapers, you have cause for concern. Some women do have primary supply problems, as opposed to "demand" supply problems, when a baby is nursing less frequently than he should, but almost always those problems can be solved. Supplementing with formula should be a last resort, although it's necessary if your baby needs nourishment. Breastfeeding advocates would look askance at giving a young baby a bottle: A baby with feeding difficulties almost certainly will have nipple confusion. (It's easier to bottlefeed than to breastfeed, as babies quickly learn.)

Try to drink more liquids—water and juice, not commercial

sodas, because the caffeine can affect your milk—as well as an herbal remedy called Mother's Milk Tea. Although in the United States, there is only anecdotal support for herbal milk supply boosters, many moms report good results from taking blessed thistle as well as fenugreek; ask a lactation consultant to help you resolve the feeding difficulties and help with an herbal program.

See also Fenugreek; Herbal Remedies and Supplements, About; Mother's Milk Tea; Nipple Confusion; Weight Gain and Newborns

Milk: Overabundant Supply

Q: My breasts get so engorged that milk literally squirts out of the nipples. They look like little fire hoses. My daughter's mouth gets so full that she dribbles when she suckles for the first few minutes, and my other nipple drips so heavily that it soaks two thick cloth diapers. Is this normal? How can I slow the letdown?

A: Too much of a good thing is a problem that other moms wish they had. You can tame an overenthusiastic letdown by pumping or hand-expressing for 2 or 3 minutes before you put your baby to the breast.

See also Cabbage Leaves and Engorged Breasts; Overactive Letdown

Miscarriage and Milk Production

Q: I had a miscarriage late in my pregnancy, but my breasts are still producing milk. I tried to give some milk to a local hospital, but they said they can't take it. How can I stop lactating?

A: Our condolences on your loss.

One alternative, if you're willing to pump, is donating to a human milk bank. (*See* Milk, Donating.) Most milk banks are desperate for donor milk, especially for premature babies. Your contribution would be a wonderful way to help other families, and it may help ease some of your pain.

There's no one-size-fits-all answer for your question. Lactation ceases at different rates for different women, and some women continue until they reach menopause.

If you're painfully engorged, you can use cold cabbage leaf compresses and cold packs to relieve pain and swelling. A supportive sports bra may help you feel more comfortable. Do not bind your breasts—binding can cause a plugged duct. You can hand-express or pump a little milk if you're extremely engorged. (Don't worry—this won't increase your milk supply.)
See also Cabbage Leaves; Engorged Breasts; Appendix

Mother's Milk Tea

Q: What is Mother's Milk Tea? Does it work?

A: Some women swear by Mother's Milk Tea as a supply-booster; others can drink it by the gallon with no noticeable result. It's also inappropriate for diabetic women, who should avoid fenugreek. Many lactation consultants advise their clients to use a fenugreek tincture rather than the tea, because it's difficult to find ingredients fresh enough to be effective and because you need to drink a lot of the tea in order to see an effect. There are various commercial versions of Mother's Milk Tea, and many home recipes. Almost all variations include fenugreek and blessed thistle. (If the tea includes fenugreek, your urine and sweat may smell like maple syrup.)

If you want to make your own, here's one recipe:

Mother's Milk Tea
3 oz fennel seed
3 oz anise seed
3 oz caraway seed
1½ oz cracked fenugreek seed
1½ oz blessed thistle
1½ oz chocolate mint

Mix and store in a mason jar. Use a heaping tablespoon to a quart of water to make tea. Steep for about 5 minutes. The chocolate mint is added as a sweet flavoring, not as a supply-booster; without the mint, this is a somewhat bitter tea.
See also Appendix

Multiples, Nursing

See Tandem Nursing

N

Night Nursing and Babies' Teeth

Q: Does night nursing lead to decayed teeth in infants who've already started teething? My sister-in-law said that even breastfed babies can have "bottle-rot" tooth decay.

A: Opinions vary, but there is little medical evidence on which factors contribute to dental caries ("bottle rot" or nursing caries) in toddlers and very young children. Only a small percentage of breastfed babies develop dental caries while breastfeeding. Dental caries are rare in babies and young children. The La Leche League in an April 1994 statement contended that dental caries occur despite breastfeeding, not because of it.

Medical reports suggest that tooth decay is far more common in formula-fed babies, particularly those who've taken a bottle of formula or juice to bed. Dental caries are caused by nearly any liquid, apart from water, that pools in an infant's mouth for a long time. (Breast milk is swallowed as soon as the baby elicits it, without leaving a puddle of liquid in the baby's mouth.) When teeth bask in a sugary liquid, bacteria in the mouth changes the sugars to the acids that attack tooth enamel.

Dental caries can occur in a breastfed baby if the baby co-sleeps with her mother and keeps the nipple in her mouth for long periods of time. Sufficient milk will leak from the nipple to start the process that transforms milk sugars to acids.

The best solution is prevention. Keep your baby's mouth clean. Rub her gums with a clean, damp washcloth after feedings and before bedtime. Once the baby is teething, brush her teeth at least once a day with a soft infant toothbrush. A plain

washcloth or toothbrush is fine up to about age 3, when you can introduce fluoride toothpaste.
See also Teething and Nursing

Nipple Blanching

Q: After every feeding, my right nipple loses its color—the tip turns purple or white—and tingles painfully. The nipple actually contracts involuntarily, as though it's cold, and it can't relax. This lasts about 30 minutes. Then it's OK again until the next feeding. None of the other moms I know have experienced this. Is it unusual? What should I do about it?

A: Nipple blanching, also known as Reynaud's syndrome of the nipple, or vasoconstriction, is fairly common, especially if your baby tends to chomp down when he's nursing. Symptoms can appear during pregnancy and continue after the baby is born, or they can appear as a response to nipple trauma or pain. In some women, vasoconstriction occurs before and during feedings as well as afterward. The syndrome is an autoimmune response to nipple damage. Basically, the veins in your nipples contract as if they're reacting to pain or extreme cold.

Trauma and nipple pain are the most common cause, but a study cited in the *Breastfeeding Review* (May 1996) suggested that vasoconstriction is more likely to occur in women who smoke two or more cigarettes a day, or drink more than 8 ounces of coffee or other caffeinated drinks. It's also associated with allergies and with certain medications, including theophylline and terbutaline.

If your case is caused by nipple trauma—your baby chomps down in response to an overactive letdown, or is incorrectly latching on, for example—then you need a lactation consultant's help to diagnose the nursing problem and fix it. If the cause is something else, heat will help. Before and after nursing, ease the pain with warm compresses—the warmer, the better. (Nipple blanching tends to be more severe if you're chilled.) Try half-filling a cotton sock with dry rice, microwaving it for a minute, and pressing it against your nipples after a feed. (Cover your skin with a cloth diaper or burp rag if the sock is uncomfortably warm. Or use a hot-water bottle.)

If heat doesn't help, try a topical nitroglycerin paste; ask your lactation consultant to show you how to use it. Some women find that the pain is eased by the herbal supplements flax/borage oil, or evening primrose/fish oil. Moderate aerobic exercise—a brisk walk around the neighborhood, or parking a block or two farther from work—will help, too.

If the condition still persists, see your doctor, and ask about Nifedipine, a prescription drug that works as a calcium channel blocker and is compatible with breastfeeding.

Sometimes this condition is related to thrush. If you have other symptoms, treat accordingly.

See also Lactation Consultant; Nipple Pain, About; Overactive Letdown

Nipple, Bleeding

Q: My 3-week-old son has a tremendously strong suck and now a case of thrush. I'm not sure which is causing my nipple to bleed when I pump milk. How can I stop the bleeding?

A: When you say that your little guy has a strong suck, do you mean that his sucking is painful when you nurse? After the first week or so of nursing, breastfeeding should not still be painful. If it is, something is wrong that should be corrected. There may be a problem with his latch-on, or with the positioning during nursing, that is causing nipple trauma.

It's possible that your nipple was damaged before you started pumping, and now that your son has thrush, that's contributing to the bleeding and trauma. (A traumatized nipple is fertile ground for a thrush infection; it's smart to treat yourself as well as the baby for thrush. Otherwise, you can continue to pass a fungal infection back and forth.) Treating the thrush will help resolve the bleeding and soreness.

Your pump may also be contributing to the problem. Cheap, poorly made pumps can damage sensitive nipple tissue. Even a

good hospital-grade pump can damage your nipples if you're not careful about positioning the flanges and conscientious about varying the suction pressure.
See also Pumping, About; Thrush, About

Nipple Blister

Q: I had very sore nipples during my baby's first month of nursing, but then all was well until today. One nipple is very painful and has what looks like a pimple or blister on one side. Should I see a doctor?
A: It sounds like a bleb, a white spot that usually accompanies a plugged duct. There are some home techniques that help clear a plugged duct, but if it develops into mastitis, you will need to see your doctor.
See also Bleb; Milk Blisters; Mastitis, About; Plugged Ducts, About

Nipple Confusion

Q: I think my newborn has nipple confusion. At the hospital, the nurses gave him a couple of bottles. When I try to nurse him, he either doesn't open his mouth wide enough, or gives up after a few moments if he does latch on. I've been pumping and feeding him expressed milk, but I'd rather nurse.
A: Sometimes it takes babies a long time to figure out that the breast is a useful thing. And if they've had bottles, especially bottles that use preemie nipples with three holes instead of one, they tend to be discouraged by how much harder it is to get breast milk. (Other factors, including texture and taste, contribute to nipple confusion as well.) Babies who have been bottle-fed for the first 2 weeks of life often refuse to breastfeed, even if the mother has an abundant supply of milk.

Some techniques to try:

- Express a little milk, by hand or with your breast pump, so you're getting a letdown before the baby latches on. A baby who's used to the bottle may be frustrated that the breast doesn't yield milk instantaneously, as a bottle does, and expressing a little milk will jump-start the nursing session. The taste and scent of fresh milk on your nipple will encourage him to latch on. (This trick also works if you're so engorged that the baby can't get a grip on your nipple.) Breast compression while you're nursing helps, too (*see* Breast Compression).

- Use nipples with only one hole, so the baby has to work harder at the bottle. It will take much longer to get through a bottle feed, but this also eases the transition to breastfeeding.
- Attempt to latch the baby on only when the baby is relaxed, not when he's so hungry that he's too frantic to nurse. Watch for early signs—rooting around, opening and closing his mouth, etc.—that he's hungry.
- Have a lactation consultant or doula watch a nursing session or two. She can help correct any problems.

See also Finger Feeding; Lactation Consultant

Nipple, Cracked

Q: I am nursing my 4-week-old son, and my left nipple is cracked. It is very painful to nurse on that side. I've used both vitamin E oil and lanolin for 5 days, but neither seems effective. What can I do?

A: A cracked nipple usually is due to a problem with positioning and latch-on. Cracks are not normal. Where the crack (or cracks) is located often indicates the problem's source. You're smart to continue to nurse from the affected nipple: Studies show that a cracked nipple heals just as quickly if it's used for nursing as if it's left alone. Nursing may speed healing, since it increases the blood flow to your breasts.

To promote healing, apply breast milk to the nipple cracks, and let it air-dry. Breast milk not only will heal cracks better than lanolin, vitamin E, or other creams but also can prevent infections. You'll also need an all-purpose nipple ointment to heal a damaged nipple, and moist wounds require special care. Ask your doctor or lactation consultant for help.

First, check your baby when she's off the breast, and see if she can extend her tongue beyond her gum line. If she can't extend her tongue, that might be the cause of your cracked nipple. Have your pediatrician look at her tongue to confirm this. It's possible to breastfeed in this case, but you'll need one-to-one help from a lactation consultant who's had experience with this situation.

If your cracked nipple was caused by a positioning problem, here are some tips on establishing a good nursing position:

- Have several small pillows available to support your arms and your baby. Nurse in a comfortable chair, or surround yourself with pillows if you're nursing in bed. Put one pillow behind your back, another on your lap, and a third under the arm that you'll use to support the baby.
- Rest your feet on a low footstool (a cardboard box will work in a pinch), so your knees are raised.
- Hold the baby at breast level. The pillows should be supporting your upper body—arms and shoulders—and your lower back. If those areas feel strained, reposition yourself.
- Check the baby to make sure she also feels supported and secure. If she's tense, she can't concentrate on nursing.
- Hold your breast with one hand. Cup it with your thumb above—but not touching—the pink/brown areola, so your fingers and palm support the breast from below. Tickle your baby's lips with your nipple. If she doesn't open her lips, express a little milk and dab it on her mouth. When she opens her mouth, bring her quickly to your breast.
- Make sure she gets a big mouthful of breast. Your whole nipple should be inside her mouth, and a good measure (an inch) of areola as well. (If you're engorged, you may not be able to get much or any areola inside. Express some milk until the engorgement diminishes.)

- Support the baby, if necessary, at her shoulders, instead of her head. Make sure her body is in a straight line from ear to hip. Cuddle her close. Her chin and nose should be in contact with your breast throughout the session.
- Watch her as she suckles. Are her lips pulled in, or flanged out? If they're pulled in, fold the lip out. If you're having trouble envisioning this, watch yourself in the mirror while you're drinking a soda from a can or bottle. That's how the baby's lips should look, too.
- Listen as she nurses. If she clicks, slurps, or gasps, she may have a poor latch-on.

See also Breast Compression; Latching On, About; Positions, About; Palate, High; Cleft Lip; Nipple Ointment; Nipples, Sore, About

Nipple Damage

Q: A few days ago, my 6-month-old bit my nipple, breaking the skin. I'm having trouble nursing on that breast because the wound keeps reopening. Should I stop nursing on that side?

A: You may want to ease off nursing on that side for a few days, but don't stop completely. (Your breast will be painfully engorged, and you risk infection and diminished milk supply.)

Have you tried using ointments to promote healing? Over-the-counter cortisone cream, applied after each nursing session, should help. If the ointments don't help, you should see your OB/GYN to make sure that something else is not hampering the healing.

Nipple Discharge

See Bloody Nipple Discharge; Rusty Pipe Syndrome

Nipple Ointment

Q: I've been breastfeeding for 4 weeks, gritting my teeth because my nipples are sore, cracked, and excruciatingly painful. What can I do to make them feel better?

A: The best treatment is prevention: making sure that your baby has a good latch. But nipple ointments—not creams, which can dry your skin further—can help moderate pain. Many moms use Lasinoh and Purlan with good results.

If that doesn't help, talk to your OB/GYN about prescription ointments containing antibiotics. If your nipples are cracked, chances are that the cracks contain bacteria that are either delaying the healing process or augmenting an infection. Antibiotic ointments crack down on the bacteria and also alleviate pain. To use an ointment, apply a thin coat on your nipples after each feeding. Do not wipe or wash it off, even if the baby wants to nurse again in a few minutes. (The few ingredients that your baby absorbs will not harm him.) Most ointments are effective within a few days to a week. It's possible to continue using the ointments after the pain disappears, but most moms prefer to cut back or eliminate the ointment once the pain's gone.

See also Nipples, Sore, About

Nipple Pain, About

Nearly every woman who's breastfed a baby has had some nipple pain. When you're first breastfeeding, you'll probably find it painful when the baby first latches on. When your breasts are tender, even a correctly latched-on newborn's mouth can feel like a vise grip.

This is why it's so important to get a lactation consultant or a doula to watch a nursing session. She can tell if the pain is the temporary sort associated with early nursing, or if it's due to latch-on problems. If the baby is correctly latched, you should feel a slight tugging sensation, not pain.

If the pain refuses to go away, you may have a latch-on problem. It may sound like a cop-out to keep recommending lactation consultants, but: Get another lactation consultant—one who specializes in difficult nursing situations—and have her watch you during a nursing session. A good lactation consultant can mean the difference between nursing in misery and nursing in comfort. Sometimes the smallest change in nursing position will resolve the problem.

A good lactation consultant can help resolve the positioning and latch-on problems. If you stick with nursing, you'll find that with time and experience, breastfeeding will be comfortable, not painful.

Preventing and managing nipple pain:

- Let your nipples air-dry after a feeding.
- If they feel dry, clean them with water only, not soap.
- Rub expressed milk into dry, cracked, or blistered nipples, as well as an all-purpose nipple ointment.
- Use warm compresses on sore nipples.
- Watch for the warning signs of thrush—extremely pink, raw-looking nipples; plugged ducts, blisters or cracks; shiny or taut areola skin; blanched nipple tips; pain and burning between feedings—and treat promptly.
- Use a pump to express milk (and help maintain your supply) if your nipples are so sore that you can't bear to nurse.
- Monitor the suction on your breast pump. Increasing the pressure can make your nipples sore and red.
- If your nipples are sensitive only periodically, start tracking your menstrual cycle. Many nursing moms find that their nipples are hypersensitive when they're ovulating and/or about to menstruate.

See also Lactation Consultant; Nipple Blanching; Nipple Confusion; Palate, High; Pumping, About; Thrush, About; Weaning, About

Nipple Pain, Unidentifiable

Q: My 8-month-old daughter and I have struggled endlessly with thrush, so I know how to recognize and deal with it. None of the signs are there except the pain: I grimace, hiss, and curl my toes during latch-on and the first few minutes of nursing. This leaves me tired, cranky, and sore. What's going on?

A: Hmm—tired, cranky, and sore, with extremely sensitive nipples. Have you taken a pregnancy test? You could be pregnant. If you take a home pregnancy test, remember that early in pregnancy you can get false negatives. If it's not positive, and your symptoms continue, test again in a day or two.

It also is possible, given your history with thrush, that your old enemy is back. You might try gentian violet, which could help if it is thrush, and in any case won't hurt (unless you count light-colored clothing and towels). Because it works so swiftly, you'll know within a couple of days whether you're dealing with thrush or something else.

If the gentian violet is ineffective, and the pregnancy test results are negative, see your doctor.

See also Nipple Pain, About; Thrush, About

Nipple Preference

Q: I'm trying to introduce my 7-week-old son to the bottle, but I'm not having much luck. He just spits out the nipple. What should I do?

A: There's no reason to force a breastfed baby to take a bottle. Have you tried a cup? He may take more readily to a sippy cup—a cup whose spout has holes or a slit.

If you must use a bottle, try offering different kinds of artificial nipples. Just as your baby may favor one of your breasts over the other, a bottle-fed baby often prefers one artificial nipple over other brands. Avent and Evenflo are two brands that many breastfed babies accept, but you may need to keep trying until you find the one your baby will take.

See also Appendix

Nipple Shields, Baby Refuses to Nurse Without

Q: I needed to use nipple shields for the first few weeks after my son was born because my breasts were so engorged and I had inverted nipples. Now the nipples emerge enough on their own for my daughter to latch onto, but she won't nurse unless I'm wearing the shields. I'd really like to get rid of them. What should I do?

A: To wean your baby from the shield, start each feeding with the nipple shield in place. About 4 or 5 minutes into the feed, slip the shield off. Don't worry if sometimes your baby refuses to take your bare nipple. Switch breasts, and repeat the procedure. If you're persistent—first the shield, then the nipple—at each nursing session, eventually your bare breast will be preferable.

Be sure to watch your baby for signs that she's getting enough fluids: 8 to 10 wet diapers a day, and 4 or 5 bowel movements daily.

See also Breast Shells; Nipple Shields

Nipple Shields

Q: I've had problems with flat, sore nipples and a bout of mastitis in the 2 weeks since my son was born. My doctor recommended nipple shields, but my midwife advised against them. I don't want to use nipple shields unless they actually help.

A: The answer is yes, and no. A nipple shield is a silicone nipple that fits over your own. The baby actually latches onto the nipple shield, instead of your bare nipple, to nurse. (Breast shells, in contrast, are two-part devices designed to force inverted nipples to quit hiding and perk up.)

Nipple shields are a tool used temporarily to help resolve breastfeeding problems. A lactation consultant should show you how to use and care for a nipple shield, help fix the feeding problems that make it necessary, and help you wean the baby from the shield.

See also Breast Shells; Nipple Pain, About; Nipples, Inverted; Nipples, Sore, About; Plugged Ducts, About

Nipples, Droopy

Q: I'd like to breastfeed my baby, but I worry that nursing will make my breasts and nipples droop and look ugly. What effect will breastfeeding have on my nipples?

A: How do your nipples look now? Pregnancy changes breasts more than nursing. If you have flat or inverted nipples, breastfeeding will draw them out, but the change may not be permanent.

In any case, your body will change as you age, and it's inevitable that your breasts will change, too, whether you breastfeed or bottlefeed your baby. Changes during your pregnancy, and your genetic makeup—not breastfeeding—determine their appearance.

Nipples, Inverted

Q: My obstetrician told me that I have inverted nipples and that it may be difficult to breastfeed. I'm 35 weeks pregnant, and another mom told me that it might be too late to un-invert them. Is she right? What can I do?

A: Inverted or flat nipples usually are the result of the ligaments along the milk ducts, which run to the ducts and nipples, being short and a little off center. The ligaments pull in the end of the nipple, inverting it. This isn't an insurmountable problem—"most babies can suck the paint off a wall," observed one lactation consultant—but you do need time, patience, and a little technological help from a breast shell.

Skin and tissue are elastic and can be reshaped. If you grasp the nipple, you can pull it out until it protrudes. The problem is that it returns to the inverted position when you let it go.

The logic behind breast shells, or using a pump to extrude inverted nipples, is that the more often you can get the nipple to protrude, the more likely it is to remain protruded. Pull it out 100 times, and it will protrude for a while. Pull it out 1,000 times, as a breast shell does, and it may protrude permanently.

Practical ways to encourage nipples to protrude include using breast shells (two-part contraptions that gently pressure the tissue around the nipple and force it out) and using a hospital-grade breast pump. Manual pumps aren't as effective; you need something with suction strong enough to stretch out your nip-

ple and keep it stretched long enough to stretch the ligaments, too. Ask a lactation consultant for help with breast shells and to help establish breastfeeding after your baby is born.
See also Breast Shells; Nipple Shields; Pumping, About; Nipples, Sore, About

Nipples, Long

Q: I don't have large breasts, but I do have long nipples. My 6-week-old has trouble latching on—he can't get his tongue and lower lip over the areola. I've been pumping and giving him breast milk by bottle, along with nursing him. I've tried every nursing position I can think of. What else can I do?

A: Some babies have trouble latching on to long nipples. Their little mouths are so small that they can't get enough breast tissue into their mouths to compress the milk ducts. Time will help: As he gets bigger, he'll be able to take in more of the areola.

Meanwhile, get professional help. A lactation consultant can help show you how to use nipple shields and how to try different methods of latching the baby onto your breast. Among the best positions in this situation is the football hold, and it's important to really snuggle your son into your breast. Have you tried the modified football hold, with the baby on your side, sitting up so he's looking down at your breast (and not up at you)?
See also Positions, About

Nipple, Pierced

See Pierced Nipple

Nipples, Sore, About

Some mothers have sore nipples, even if their babies seem (to an untrained eye) to be properly latched on, with textbook-style suckling. Pain always indicates a problem that needs to be diagnosed and resolved.Breastfeeding is not normally a painful experience. With some detective work, you may be able to isolate the source of your pain and remedy the problem.

If you've had pain nursing right off the bat—nipple pain that hasn't lessened since your first nursing session—there may be a problem with positioning, latch-on, or your baby's suck. It also is possible that the problem is physical. Ask the pediatrician and/or your lactation consultant to examine your baby's mouth. She may have a high palate, or a short or tight frenulum (the tissue under the tongue) that makes it difficult for her to use her tongue.

If breastfeeding already is established, and your nipples are suddenly sore, you may have thrush. To properly diagnose thrush, both you and the baby should be examined by a lactation consultant and then by your physician. Sometimes, even if you've taken medication for thrush—lotrimin, loprox, nystatin—the thrush may still be present if you *and* the baby haven't been treated simultaneously for at least 2 weeks. Thrush is persistent, and it can be resistant to drugs, returning after you think that you've treated it. If you do have thrush, do *not* treat your nipples with hydrocortisone; it only makes your nipples even more sore.

If your nipples are red and sore, but thrush has been ruled out, another possibility is eczema of the nipples. This occurs in women with a history of eczema and dry, sensitive skin, and it usually is accompanied by burning and itching.

Sore, tender nipples also can signal pregnancy, especially if you're also exceptionally tired and nauseated. Could you have a breast inflammation or infection? Did you have mastitis? Even if you treat mastitis with penicillin, the drug may not have resolved the staph infection. If your pain is caused by a persistent staph infection, ask your doctor about dicloxacillin, which must be taken conscientiously for 2 weeks.

Could you have a bacterial infection in your nipples? Are they cracked and refusing to heal? Those infections are painful and can lead to a bout with thrush. (*See* Thrush, About.)

If you've eliminated infections, inflammation, thrush, and

positioning as the culprits, you should see a dermatologist familiar with breastfeeding-related problems. (Your lactation consultant, or the local La Leche League, should be able to suggest someone.)

Tips for preventing or healing sore nipples:

- Check the baby's position when she latches on. Make sure the nipple is pointing at the back of her mouth (*See* Latching on) and that she's encompassing as much of the nipple and areola in her mouth as possible.
- Make sure the baby's lower lip is flanged, not sucked into her mouth. Pull down his lower lip. You should be able to see his tongue between his lower lip and your nipple.
- Use warm compresses and expressing a little milk to soften nipples hardened by engorgement.
- Use your finger to break the baby's latch suction, rather than pulling the baby off your breast.

See also Breast Infections; Mastitis, About; Overactive Letdown; Pregnancy; Thrush, About

Nipples, Toughening

Q: My mother-in-law keeps telling me to "toughen up" my nipples so they won't be sore when my baby's born this spring. My midwife says scrubbing your nipples with a loofah or washcloth will only make them sore, not tough. Who is right?

A: Your midwife, even though your mother-in-law probably means well. You can't "toughen" nipples. Nipples should be flexible, not callused. A loofah or washcloth can't mimic a suckling baby, anyway—all that scrubbing causes only unnecessary pain.

Most of the time, sore nipples are caused by a poor latch-on, thrush, or flat or inverted nipples.

See also Latching On, About; Thrush, About

Nipples, White

See Nipple Blanching

No Milk, Newborn

Q: My daughter is 3 days old, and I have absolutely no milk or colostrum. I can't express even a drop. The nurses at the hospital insisted on giving her formula. So she's not hungry enough to nurse, even if I did have milk. What can I do?

A: If your infant is robust, start putting her on your breast immediately, as you should have been allowed to do from the moment your daughter was born. Babies benefit tremendously from even minute amounts of colostrum, and their mouths are the most efficient way of eliciting fluid from your breasts. Though it's unusual that your milk hasn't come in, sometimes it takes up to 5 days before you're actively lactating. (Babies are born padded with an extra layer of fat and fluid—that's why their birth weight can be deceptive, and why they often lose up to 10 percent of their body weight in the first postpartum days.)

How is her urine output? Is she alert or lethargic? Does she look healthy or jaundiced? If her wet diaper count is low, and she acts exceptionally listless and/or seems yellow, you will need to pump to stimulate your milk supply, and work with a lactation consultant to teach your baby to nurse. Until she perks up, you can try giving her only an ounce of formula—not a complete feed—to boost her incentive to breastfeed.

Start putting your baby on your breast to stimulate your nipples and to encourage your breasts to produce milk. Adapt Chicago's onetime voting policy—nurse early and often. (Renting a hospital-quality pump will help stimulate your milk production, too. *See* Pumping.) That means every 2 hours, aiming for 8 to 12 feedings in a 24-hour period.

Let your baby play a bit with your nipples—let her nuzzle and mouth them a little, to get familiar. She may be a little reluctant to breastfeed—it's much easier to get liquid from a bottle. Have a lactation consultant watch you during your first nursing sessions. She can make sure the baby's latched on, and give you hands-on assistance.

With persistence on your part and hers, your milk will come in. She'll be nursing like a champ by the time she's a month old, and formula will be a thing of the past.

See also Latching On, About; Nipple Confusion; Positions, About

No Milk?

Q: I've been nursing with no problem for several months, but last night my breasts didn't seem to produce much milk. I no longer feel the letdown, and it's been a while since I've been able to tell whether a breast is full by hoisting it in my palm. I haven't changed my diet, and the baby is nursing normally. What's going on?

A: It's most likely that you're still producing milk, since the baby is still nursing without complaint. After about 3 months, lactating breasts no longer are huge and full before a feeding session. They still produce milk, though.

If you're exclusively breastfeeding and your milk supply does diminish, it's due to other factors. Pregnancy, stress, menstruation, and certain medications, including some forms of birth control, can reduce your output. Spontaneously drying up—losing all your milk—is extremely unlikely. Usually, a change in letdown and supply is related to stress or to consumption of a dehydrating product, like coffee, caffeinated sodas, or antihistamines and cold remedies.

See also Birth Control; Herbal Remedies and Supplements, About; Resuming Menstruation, About; Pregnancy; Supply Problems, About

Nonfat Milk for Nursing Mothers

Q: Should I drink 2 percent or whole milk instead of nonfat milk? My mom says the baby needs the extra fat. I don't need the calories—I'm trying to cut down, but not if it prevents my 3-month-old daughter from getting the nutrition she needs.

A: Feel free to drink nonfat milk. A bonus: Nonfat milk has more calcium than 1 percent, 2 percent, or whole milk. Your body makes the perfect milk for your baby, no matter whether you're drinking nonfat or malted milk. If you're dieting, make sure that your choices are well balanced and that you drink plenty of water. And remember: Some of the weight you gained during pregnancy is intended for stores that will be mobilized when you lactate. (Too bad for moms who don't breastfeed—they have a harder time losing that weight.)

See also Weight Loss

Nonstop Nursing

See Cluster Feeding; Growth Spurts, About; Teething and Nursing

Nursing Bras, About

Nursing bras are immensely practical for a breastfeeding mother, especially one who is well endowed. Nursing bras also are immense, period. Few articles of clothing this side of a Wagner opera look as formidable and indestructible as the average nursing bra. But you'll be snapping it open and shut six to a dozen times a day—more during growth spurts—so indestructibility has its advantages. Most breastfeeding moms consider nursing bras indispensable, and most of us need the support that a good nursing bra offers.

For a proper fit, you'll have to wait until about 6 weeks after the baby is born. Pay no attention to the books and experts who advise you to start out with six or seven nursing bras. Your breast size will change so much during the first few weeks of your baby's life that those first nursing bras won't fit once your milk supply is established.

Instead, buy one or two nursing bras to get through the first couple of weeks. Your cup size almost certainly will change from what it was during pregnancy—but you won't know how much larger it will be until you and the baby establish a nursing routine. If you're pinched financially, use a sleep bra or a maternity bra until you can buy a good nursing bra.

When you do buy a nursing bra, don't cheap out. An inexpensive nursing bra that doesn't fit correctly will only lead to plugged ducts, mastitis, and back pain. Spend a little more money, and go to a maternity or bra specialty store that employs a bra fitter. (Or you can buy custom-made bras through Decent Exposures and other online nursing bra manufacturers.)

The fitter should measure you to determine the right bra size, and offer a choice of several different bras. Buy the one that feels the most comfortable. Bring the baby along—most stores that sell nursing bras are baby-friendly, and many have a rocking chair for nursing sessions. And you'll get a chance to test-drive your new bra.

Try out the snaps or clips, one-handed, to make sure that you'll have fairly easy access to your breasts. It's true that most nursing bras, like bicycle shorts, are as ugly as they are functional. A nursing bra looks like Soviet architecture, not Victoria's Secret. However, if you want to avoid the standard three-hook, industrial-white model, options exist.

Decent Exposures, Bravado! Designs, Leading Lady, and Olga all make nursing bras available in patterns and colors. Decent Exposure's custom-made bras are especially popular with hard-to-fit women; they come in sizes from 28AAA to 56H. You can order those bras through company Web sites (*see* Appendix) if they're unavailable at local maternity stores.

A word of warning: Resist the temptation to save money by dyeing a white nursing bra. One mom who tried it discovered that the bra took the dye—but it only took a leak or two to stain her breasts the same color.

See also Appendix

Nursing Bras and Breast Size

Q: Before I was pregnant, I wore a 36B. After nursing two children, I have a stockpile of worn but reliable nursing bras. Now, with my third child, my breasts have ballooned to Partonesque proportions. She's only 3 weeks old, and I've had to buy two new (huge) nursing bras. Will my ta-tas be this bodacious as long as I'm nursing?

A: Nursing bras are more expensive than standard bras, so your dismay is understandable. Remember that a new lactating mother's breasts tend to be the largest during the newborn's first 6 weeks. After that, as your breasts establish their milk production they should settle into a predictable size. Your bra size may be larger than before, but don't be surprised if you go down a cup size after 6 months and after weaning. It can take a year or more after weaning before your breasts return to their true size—and that may be a bit larger than your prepregnancy size, or it may be smaller. One mom went from a 36C before pregnancy to 32A after her last child weaned.

See also Nursing Bras, About

Nursing Constantly

Q: My 5-week-old baby nurses virtually nonstop at night. She'll nurse, latch off, and then want to nurse again 5 or 10 minutes later. Is this normal? I feel as if all I do is nurse 24 hours a day! My mother wants me to give her rice cereal. Isn't she awfully young for solids?

A: What you're describing is very common, especially with a baby that age. They can be real barnacles for the first month or so! Milk supply is typically lower in the evenings, and infants like to nurse to wind down at night.

As you guessed, a 5-week-old's digestive system is too immature for solids. Even if she managed to get any down, she'd just be up all night with an aching tummy—her digestive system is too immature to handle solids.

Try sleeping with her, in your bed. That way, she can latch on and off, and you'll be resting as well without having to get up and down all night.

Nursing Constantly and Slow Weight Gain

Q: My 9-week-old daughter is fussy all the time. She wants to be nursed or carried nonstop. She sleeps for 3 to 4 hours at night, but never longer than 30 minutes during the day. Even with all the nursing, she's not gaining enough weight. How can I keep her calm and get her to gain some weight?

A: A 9-week-old baby who is not gaining weight appropriately should be seen immediately by your pediatrician. A lactation consultant should visit you and observe a feeding session to diagnose possible latching difficulties or other problems.

See also Baby Carriers, About; Colic; Diaper Count; Foremilk and Hindmilk; Weight Gain, Slow; Appendix

Nursing Frequently, Older Baby

Q: My 5-month-old baby usually sleeps all night, but suddenly yesterday and today he wanted to nurse every 2 hours, all day and all night. What's going on?

A: He may be starting to teethe. Some babies find that suckling helps relieve the pressure and pain of teeth cutting through the gums. Or he may be among the babies who start changing their nighttime sleep patterns when they reach 5 to 7 months. Or he may be hungry, and ready for solid foods (which will help him sleep for longer stretches).

Other possibilities:

- He may be hitting his 6-month growth spurt a little early.
- He may be reaching a developmental milestone. Is he starting to sit up alone, roll over, babble?
- He may have separation anxiety.
- He may have an ear infection: Some babies suckle to relieve the pressure in their ears. (Watch for a fever, a runny nose, fretfulness, or distress, especially at naptime and bedtime.)

If he's going through a growth spurt or a developmental milestone, his nursing needs should slow down, and his sleeping pattern resume, in a few days. If not, try introducing solid foods.

Nursing Multiples

See Tandem Nursing

Nursing Pads

Q: Can you tell me where to find reusable cotton nursing pads? I don't like the disposable kind.

A: Cotton nursing pads are available in some department stores, including JC Penney, and at some drug stores, including Osco Pharmacy. Most stores that sell nursing bras and maternity products also sell nursing pads, or you can check in baby product catalogues and through online baby product Web sites. Among the names to seek out: Born To Love, a natural baby product catalog; Motherwear (online at www.motherwear.com); Medela; Milk Diapers; Natural Baby; online through Mother's Nature, www.babyholder.com; and through www.childsecure.com.

Remember: Cotton pads, like cotton diapers, need to be washed frequently. If you're engorged, or if your supply is ample, you'll need to double up on the number of pads you use—and even then, you still might leak through.

Nursing in Public

See Breastfeeding in Public, About

Nursing Station

Q: How do you set up a nursing station?

A: A nursing station is just an area where you can comfortably nurse without having to get up in the middle of the session for a glass of water or new pillows.

Your nursing station should include a table and a comfortable chair. Keep a pitcher of water and a glass on the table, plus snacks you can eat one-handed, and—if you're dextrous, a slender magazine or a paperback novel. (If you can read and breastfeed simultaneously, it's a lot easier to get through the marathon nursing sessions associated with growth spurts, teething, and ear infections.)

Most moms like recliners or rocking chairs, but you can use any chair that gives you adequate back support and is wide enough to allow you to nurse in different positions.

Nursing Strike

Q: Help! My 4-month-old daughter refuses to nurse. I'm afraid she's going to dehydrate herself or starve. She's been erratic for 20 hours—she either won't latch on at all, or releases only a minute or two after starting to nurse. I hate to force her, but I'm worried about her health and about my milk drying up because she won't nurse.

A: She may be reacting to a change in you. Consider some common factors that lead to (usually temporary) nursing strikes:

- Your period returns or you're pregnant (hormonal changes affect the milk's taste).
- She has an ear infection.
- There's been a change in routine.
- She's teething.
- She bit you, and your reaction frightened her.
- She's distracted (especially if she's an older baby).

Every baby is different. Don't take the rejection personally. Keep watching the baby. When she seems hungry, put her back to your breast. Express a little milk and rub it on her lips. If you're painfully engorged, pump some milk. Be patient.

Try taking her into a dark, quiet room to nurse. If you can, choose a time of day when she traditionally nurses longer—before naptime or bedtime, for example. Some babies will nurse if you sit with them in a warm bath.

Does she have a fever? Sometimes teething babies run a slight fever. Ear infections are usually accompanied by a fever and by restless sleep (waking every hour or so). Consult your pediatrician if she's running a fever or if her nursing pattern continues to be erratic. Make sure you count the number of wet diapers she produces—put a tissue between her bottom and the diaper if you use disposables—to make sure she's not dehydrated.

Don't worry about how much milk your breasts are producing. The supply will match demand if your baby resumes nursing. (If your baby doesn't nurse regularly, your supply may drop and not be adequate for your baby's needs.) If you're uncomfortably engorged, pump milk at feeding times.

See also Dehydration; Engorged Breasts; Pumping, About

Nursing Strike, or Weaning?

Q: My 9-month-old daughter has decided that she's finished breastfeeding. She still takes a bottle of expressed milk from Dad, with no problem. This is her third day of not nursing at all. The first day, she didn't nurse at all after she fell and hurt her lip. Then she nursed twice on the second day, and so far not at all today. Could she be weaning herself, or is this a nursing strike? I'm tired of trying to force her to nurse, and I'm worried about a breast infection: I'm so full of milk that I'm ready to explode.

A: This sounds like a strike. First, pump your breasts several times a day. That will relieve your engorgement and keep up your supply when your daughter returns to nursing. (If you don't pump, your milk will start to change its taste, as it does when you're deliberately weaning.)

Sounds as if you're doing the right thing by offering gently and frequently. Some unselfconscious moms even go around topless to encourage nursing. You might also try a family bed—sleeping with your daughter in your bed—to encourage her to nurse at night; a baby sometimes nurses more readily when she's sleepy than when she's awake.

Nursing strikes rarely last more than a few days, although

some last longer. One little boy broke his tooth, and his nursing strike lasted more than 3 weeks—which was how long it took to get a dentist to treat the tooth. With an exposed nerve, the boy was in too much pain to suckle. Once your daughter's lip heals, she'll probably be interested in nursing again.
See also Weaning, About

Nursing and Teething

Q: My 7-month-old is working on her second tooth. She won't take a bottle or a pacifier, although she will drink from a sippy cup. She nurses frequently when she's teething. Sometimes I'm up every hour or two with her. I know she'll grow out of this, but I'm delirious from sleep deprivation. How can I keep her from using me as a teether instead of as a food source?

A: There's no magic cure, but you can try some things to distract her:

- Lots of walks and daily trips out
- A wet or frozen washcloth to teethe on
- A frozen bagel or corn cob (corn kernels removed) to chew on, if she's taking solids
- A plastic-tipped baby spoon to teethe on, between meals
- A hard teething biscuit, available in supermarkets and health food stores
- Orajel or infant Tylenol on her gums

See also Biting, About; Teething and Nursing

Nursing Tops

Q: I'm expecting a baby in 2 months, and I intend to breastfeed. Are special nursing shirts worth the money? They don't look that different from giant T-shirts, and most of the ones I've seen are unattractive.

A: Some moms prefer nursing shirts, especially when they're away from home, because the shirts are designed for maximum coverage while breastfeeding. Some nursing tops aren't much more than a T-shirt with a fold or two of fabric to cover the slits over your breasts. Other (higher-priced) versions are so tailored that you have to look twice to see that they're nursing tops.

You often can find nursing tops in secondhand shops that specialize in baby and maternity clothing and products. You may want to buy one to see if you like it. A nursing top can help you feel more self-assured about breastfeeding in public. A word of advice: Avoid the tops with diagonally placed flaps if you live in a breezy area. A wind gust can flip up one of the folds meant to cover your nursing bra.

If you don't like nursing tops, you can just wear loose-fitting T-shirts, with a button-front vest, jacket, or shirt for extra coverage in cool temperatures.

See also Appendix

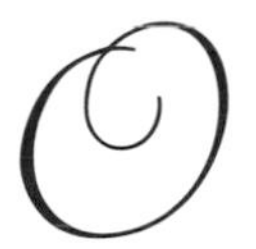

"Off" Smell in Expressed Milk

See Lipase, Excess; Pumping, About

Otitis Media (Middle Ear Infection)

See Ear Infection

Overactive Letdown

Q: My milk lets down so fast that sometimes it sprays my newborn daughter's face, and she has to gulp to keep up with the flow. She gets so much milk from one breast that usually she's not interested in nursing on the other one. She's very fussy, and full of burps and flatulence, which make her so uncomfortable that she rarely sleeps more than 10 to 45 minutes. I'm exhausted and so is she. What can I do?

A: Sounds as if you have the classic case of overactive letdown. Some moms have supply problems; others, like you, have too much milk. Your daughter's gassiness is caused by swallowing a lot of air as she tries to keep up with the milk flow and the overabundance of foremilk that she's probably getting. (Does she tend to have green stools?) Foremilk is high in lactose, which causes gas.

Signs of overactive letdown include

- A fussy, gassy baby
- Milk that squirts out so fast that the baby either struggles to swallow, or pulls away and lets the milk spray
- Sympathetic letdown in the unused breast during nursing sessions

Most babies eventually learn how to keep up with the flow of milk, and your breast milk production will adjust to her needs. Some ways to help her (and you) cope:

- If she's pulling away while she's nursing, let her off while you express some milk to slow the flow. Relatch her after your milk stops spraying.
- If she nurses and gulps, interrupt the feed every 4 or 5 minutes to burp her. That will help with the gas.
- Nurse her on one breast per feeding, or on the same breast for 2 hours or more, until she empties it. This makes sure she gets both the watery, lactose-heavy foremilk and the creamier, caloric hindmilk.
- Forget about timing your feeds to last only a fixed period of time. Let your daughter decide when she's finished, instead of taking her off your breast. She may be finished in less than 5 minutes, or she may nurse for 45 minutes. (Don't worry: This won't last forever. It just seems that way.)
- Alternate breasts at each feeding. (With an overactive letdown, it's usually easy to tell which breast wasn't nursed—it's another cup size larger!)

Don't worry if your daughter drools a little milk (a few drops or so) while she nurses, or if she spits up a bit when you burp her after a feeding. Many babies spit up after feeds (breast milk or formula) for the first 6 months. You'll know that your daughter is getting enough milk if she is gaining weight, is alert and happy, and produces plenty of wet and poopy diapers.

See also Diaper Count; Pulling on Nipple

Overfeeding

Q: I don't understand why people say you can't overfeed a breastfed baby, when it's possible to overfeed a bottle-fed baby. Does it have to do with how easily breast milk is digested?

A: Actually, it's the sucking–nipple combination that makes the difference. When a baby drinks from a bottle, the liquid from the nipple continues to flow whether she sucks or not. It's a choice of swallow or drown.

But when a baby nurses at the breast, the milk won't flow after the first minute or so of letdown unless the baby is actively suckling. Most babies learn during the first 3 to 6 weeks of life how to suckle at the breast without actually drawing much milk. This is called nonnutritive sucking. Babies like to do this for comfort.

The same logic applies when you consider nighttime nursing. A breastfed baby is less likely than a bottle-fed baby to develop caries ("bottle mouth"). If a baby falls asleep at the breast, the milk stops flowing. But if a baby falls asleep with the bottle in her mouth, liquid still drips from the nipple into her mouth and pools there. That leads to tooth decay and also to ear infections.

See also Night Nursing and Babies' Teeth

Ovulation While Breastfeeding

Q: I breastfeed my 5-month-old daughter about five times a day, and I haven't resumed my menstrual cycle yet. However, I've noticed the sort of egg-white mucus discharge that used to precede my period. Could I be ovulating, even though I'm not menstruating?

A: Some women do ovulate as you describe, especially when they're still nursing. Nursing five times a day is not enough to let you rely exclusively on breastfeeding as birth control. You can be ovulating—you can even be pregnant—before getting your first postpartum period. Unless you want to be pregnant right away, it's time to consider what birth control to use.
See also Birth Control, About

Oxytocin
See Letdown, Stimulating

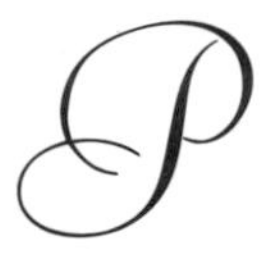

Pacifiers
Q: My son was born 5 weeks prematurely and has a weak suck. He's also been a sleepy baby. Needless to say, we've had some trouble getting him to breastfeed. My mom suggested giving him a pacifier to improve his suck, but wouldn't that create nipple confusion?
A: Generally, lactation consultants advise against introducing a pacifier before a baby is 6 to 8 weeks old, and some tell their clients not to use pacifiers at all. Babies may suck the pacifier when they need to nurse, and it can be hard, especially for a new parent, to distinguish when a baby needs to suck for food rather than for comfort. And if you're concerned about your milk supply, even nonnutritive suckling will stimulate your breasts to make more milk.

Your best recourse is to consult a lactation consultant who has had extensive experience with premature babies (ask your pedi-

atrician or the local La Leche League representative for recommendations), and work with her.
See Appendix

Pads, Nursing

See Nursing Pads

Paladai

Q: My son can't make his lips form a seal around my nipples, so even though he's trying to breastfeed, hardly any milk makes it into his stomach. An Indian friend told me to use a paladai, but my lactation consultant's never heard of this. What is it, and where can I find one?

A: A paladai is a stainless steel cup with a narrow, grooved spout. Originally, it was used to burn oil during religious ceremonies in South India, but a paladai can also be used as an infant feeding device. The All-India Institute of Medical Science in New Delhi uses the paladai in its neonatal intensive care unit to feed premature and low-birthweight babies. The paladai is also being used in clinical trials studying its effectiveness at teaching hospitals, including Pennsylvania Hospital, in the United States. As an infant feeding aid, the paladai is used only rarely in this country. Not all Indian markets carry paladais, and even if you find one, it will be difficult to track down a lactation consultant who can show you how to use it. You'd probably be better off using a more conventional alternative feeding aid.
See also Finger Feeding; Palate, High; Tube Feeding Lactation Aid

Palate, Cleft

See Cleft Lip and Breastfeeding

Palate, High

Q: My 2-week-old baby has a high palate. It's not a cleft palate—the roof of her mouth is so high that she can't get my nipple up against it. I'd like to breastfeed her, but my efforts only leave both of us mad and frustrated.

A: High palates don't get as much press as cleft palates, which also present unique nursing problems. She may grow into her palate over time. Some babies do better with short-term pumping and cup-, finger-, or bottlefeeding; ask your lactation consultant which method might work best with your baby.

Some babies with high palates have been successfully fed using a finger feeder (the Medela Hazelbaker finger feeder is a good one) to get the baby suckling, and then have made the transition to a bottle.

"Our advice is: Don't make the breast a battleground," advises the father of an infant with a high palate. His wife pumped for a month. Then they began teaching the baby to go from the bottle to the breast. By the time she was 2-1/2 months old, she was breastfeeding exclusively. (Now their problem is persuading the baby to use a bottle when the mom needs a break!)

To successfully feed her (bottle or breast), you must teach your daughter to open her mouth really wide. Ever see a picture of a snake swallowing an egg? You'll be shooting for that. With that high palate, she—and you—will need help with specific positioning and latch-on. One problem for some bottle-fed babies making the transition to breastfeeding is that the rigid bottle nipple may reshape the roof of the baby's mouth, exacerbating the problem instead of allowing it to improve.

One trick is to wait a beat or two after she opens her mouth, keeping the nipple just out of her lips' reach, until she opens just a little wider. Then, quickly, put the nipple in her mouth. You need to be fast, or she'll start closing up again. After a few days of this, she'll learn to open wider and wider, and the feeding sessions (breast or bottle) will get easier.

Hire a lactation consultant to help you through this process. With practice, determination, and a sense of humor, you'll be able to nurse.

See also Cleft Lip and Breastfeeding; Finger Feeding; Tube Feeding Lactation Aid

Permanent, Hair

Q: I didn't get a perm while I was pregnant, but now that my son is a month old, I'd like to perk up my hairstyle. Is it OK to get a perm when you're breastfeeding? Can the chemicals somehow get into the breast milk?

A: There's no danger of the permanent chemicals leaching into your milk. The only dangers are to your wallet and your morale. Since your hormones are still out of whack, you may be wasting your money on a perm. Other moms who've had perms shortly after their babies were born reported that their perms didn't last as long as usual. You might want to wait 3 or 4 months before investing in a perm.

Phentermine

Q: My baby is 5 months old, and I still weigh as much as I did when she was born. I want to go on an appetite suppressant to lose weight. A friend suggested phentermine—that it works wonders for short-term weight loss. I want to continue nursing, though. Is phentermine safe to take?

A: No. Phentermine should not be used by nursing mothers. Because of its small molecular weight—149—phentermine transfers easily, and in significant amounts, to breast milk. It can cause stimulation, anorexia, tremors, and other central nervous system deviations in a nursing baby. Case reports show that this drug is associated with a very small weight loss, so it's not really worth taking, anyway.

See also Weight Loss

Pierced Nipple

Q: I have pierced nipples. Do I have to remove my nipple ring in order to breastfeed my baby? Should I switch to barbells instead?

A: Take out the jewelry when you're nursing. Your baby might be able to get a good latch despite the nipple ring, but negotiating a piece of jewelry won't make breastfeeding any easier for her, and it could deform the shape of her mouth. Remember, many babies have trouble establishing a good latch on an unadorned nipple. Why create problems for yourselves? And a baby's suck can be strong enough to dislodge the jewelry—another consideration that should give you pause.

It's probably a good idea to forgo the nipple ring for the first few weeks of breastfeeding. Once you and the baby settle into predictable feeding patterns, you can replace the ring between feedings, if you wish. For more advice about pierced nipples and breastfeeding, look online for http://www.BME.FreeQ.com/pierce/08-nipple/breastfd.html

Pinworm Medication, Effect on Milk

Q: I just found out I have pinworms! Yuck! Can I safely take an over-the-counter drug like PinX to get rid of them, without affecting my 6-month-old baby?

A: Pyrantel pamoate, the anthelmintic used to treat pinworm, hookworm, and roundworm infestations, is absorbed only minimally if you take it orally. Usually, it's taken only once. Most of the medication is eliminated in your stools. Its peak level in your blood plasma (which affects your milk) usually is less than 0.05 to 0.13 micrograms per milliliter, and the peak occurs in less than 3 hours, according to Hale's *Medications and Mother's Milk.*

No data are available on pyrantel transferring to human milk, but because there's so little oral absorption, and its plasma levels are so low, its presence in breast milk is negligible. Take extra care with your hygiene while you're being treated, and the rest of your family should be checked for pinworms, too.

Plugged Ducts, About

A plugged duct usually announces itself as a painfully tender red blotch on your breast. The redness is a sign that the alveoli—the sacs that store your milk—are not being completely emptied when your baby nurses. The sac fills with milk, and the alveoli balloon to the breaking point. Untreated, the sac will become infected and develop into mastitis and, in the worst-case scenario, an abscess.

A plugged duct can also result from a poor latch-on, or when your baby always nurses in the same position. It can also be caused by a badly fitted nursing bra, by a shirt that's too tight, or by a baby carrier that cuts into your breast tissue.

Treat a plugged duct by getting the baby to nurse as frequently as possible on the affected breast. This is exactly the opposite of what you will want to do, because plugged ducts hurt. Grit your teeth and do it. Unless your baby has a poor suck, her suckling will unplug the duct more effectively than pumping or massage. When the plug emerges, your baby will either swallow it without noticing or spit it out. (It will look like either a small white clot, or a very thin noodle.)

Warning: Never use a plugged duct as a justification to wean the baby. The best treatment is to nurse (or express) long and often. (If you're lucky, the baby will be going through a growth spurt and want to nurse every hour!) If you stop nursing on the affected breast, the breast will only get larger, more painful, and inflamed. If the inflammation leads to infection, you'll need antibiotics to counter the possibility of a breast abscess. And an infected duct can lead to an abscess, which requires surgery—opening and draining the pus from the abscess. (Did you notice? The cures for each stage only get more painful!)

Tips on dealing with plugged ducts:

- Before you nurse, place a moist hot pack on the affected area for at least 60 seconds—longer, if possible. This helps dilate the milk ducts, and it feels good. You can make an inexpensive, effective heat pack by putting a cup of plain, dry white rice in a clean cotton sock and microwaving it for a minute. Place some fabric, like a cotton diaper or a towel, between the sock and your breast to avoid the possibility of a burn from the direct heat. You can reuse the rice-filled sock until the rice starts to smell burnt.

Tips on avoiding plugged ducts:

- Vary your nursing position once a day.
- Make sure the baby is properly latched on.
- Wear a properly-fitted nursing bra. Avoid underwire bras if you're prone to plugged ducts.
- Wear loose tops.
- Adjust your baby carrier as your baby grows and if it starts to feel awkward.

Plugged Ducts, Preventing

Q: I've had problems with plugged ducts seven times, including a bout with mastitis. Can you suggest how to prevent more infections?

A: A handbook from the Singapore-based Breastfeeding Mothers' Support Group offers these tips:

- Make sure your hands are always clean before handling your breast and nipples.
- Air-dry your nipples after every feed, and change wet nursing pads and bras promptly.
- Don't let your breasts become overfull.
- Watch for early signs of plugged ducts and breast infections.
- Pay attention to your overall health: Eat a nutritious diet, drink plenty of water, and rest frequently.

Another mom who's had her share of plugged ducts suggests these exercises to prevent or help drain them:

- Extend your arm horizontally at your side and swing it in a full circle, 10 times. Repeat with other arm.
- Lift your elbows to shoulder height, and press your palms and arms together in front of your face; you will look a little like an Indian dancer. Repeat 20 times.
- Bend at the waist, extend your arms, and cross your

wrists just above your knees. Raise your arms over your head, and lower them behind your back as far as possible. Repeat 20 times.

- Roll your right shoulder slowly, backwards and down, then forward and up, 10 times. Repeat with the other shoulder.

Plugged Ducts, Recurring

Q: I have a chronic problem with clogged ducts, especially on my left-hand side. (I've had full-blown mastitis three times.) My left breast usually produces more milk than the right. I want to keep nursing my 5-month-old daughter, but I'm tired of waking up every few weeks and feeling as if a horse kicked me in the breast! Is there anything I can do to prevent clogged ducts?

A: First, try to avoid constrictive clothing—tight bras, swimsuits, T-shirts.

- If you tend to carry your daughter on your left hip, the pressure of her weight against your breast could contribute to the problem; try using a sling, or pushing her in a stroller.
- If you notice that your breast is feeling tender—"as if a horse kicked me in the breast" is a pretty accurate description of developing mastitis—try taking a warm bath or shower and using your fingers to "comb" the sore area.
- Try nursing your daughter while you're in the bathtub. When you're nursing her, use the palm of your free hand to smooth a path from the armpit to the nipple of the tender breast.
- Put a small piece of raw cabbage on the left breast—use a small, warm piece of cabbage slightly larger than the affected area.
- Soak your breast in a basin of warm salt water—a half-teaspoon of salt per cup of water—about 15 minutes before you nurse.

See also Cabbage Leaves; Mastitis, About; Thrush, About

Plugged Duct; Baby Won't Nurse

Q: I think I may have developed a plugged duct, now that my 4-month-old son is sleeping nearly all night (6 hours at a stretch). It's on the underside of my left breast, but it's painful only when I touch it. My son prefers to nurse on the right breast, and now it's hard to get him to nurse on the left side at all. What should I do?

A: Try to get him to nurse on the affected breast. If he absolutely refuses, use a pump. Nursing (or pumping) will help clear the plug. Untreated, a plugged duct can develop into an abscess, which may mean weeks of antibiotics, even after the abscess heals. It can also lead to mastitis, which is painful, exhausting, and debilitating.

The best way to handle a plugged duct is to nurse on that side as often as possible. One mom who had recurring plugged duct problems found it helpful to position her baby with his lower lip in line with the lump, on the theory that his lower lip created the most suction.

See also Breast Infections; Plugged Ducts, About; Mastitis, About

Positions, About

In any position, it's important to make sure the baby is at nipple height. Bring the baby to nipple height, using pillows to help lift and support her, instead of leaning over to bring your nipple to her mouth. Bending and leaning can cause sore nipples, backaches, and other problems. It may help to support your breast with one hand, especially if you're large-breasted.

LATCHING ON

Getting the baby properly latched on is the key to nursing successfully. Especially during the first few weeks after birth, latch-on can be difficult. Expect to reposition and relatch frequently. Remember, both you and the baby are learning. Eventually, latching on will become automatic.

Some tricks for making the latch-on easier:

- Put clean, warm, damp washcloths on your nipples just before nursing to help stimulate letdown.
- To make sure you get as much areola as possible into the baby's mouth, support your breast, tickle his lips with your nipple, and guide the nipple and as much of the areola inside the instant he opens wide. Ideally, you should get all the areola in his mouth, but often that's only theoretically possible. Some women have an areola that's 5 inches wide. Instead, get as much areola in his mouth as possible, and listen for him to swallow, and then watch his diaper output.

See also Diaper Count

AUSTRALIAN HOLD

Best in family bed. Lie in bed with the baby latched onto your breast, and her feet near your ears, and her belly opposite your chin. This position works well when the baby is little.

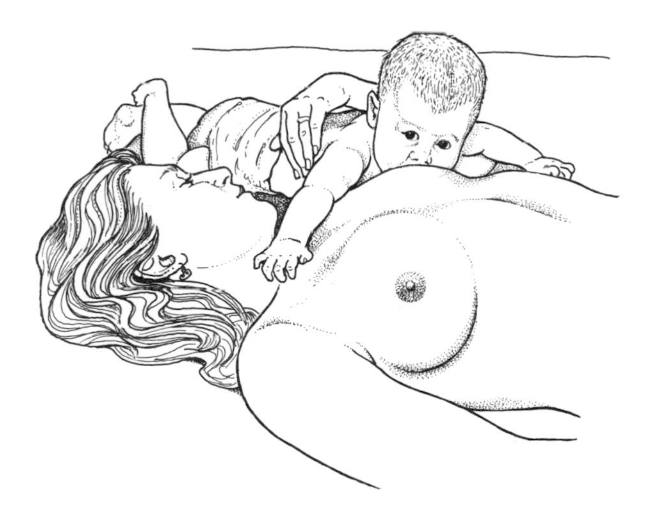

BABY UPRIGHT

Helpful for older babies who want to nurse sitting bolt upright because of congestion, reflux, or an ear infection. (Use pillows to prop babies too young to sit up on their own.) Sit the baby on your lap, facing you, and bring his head to your breast.

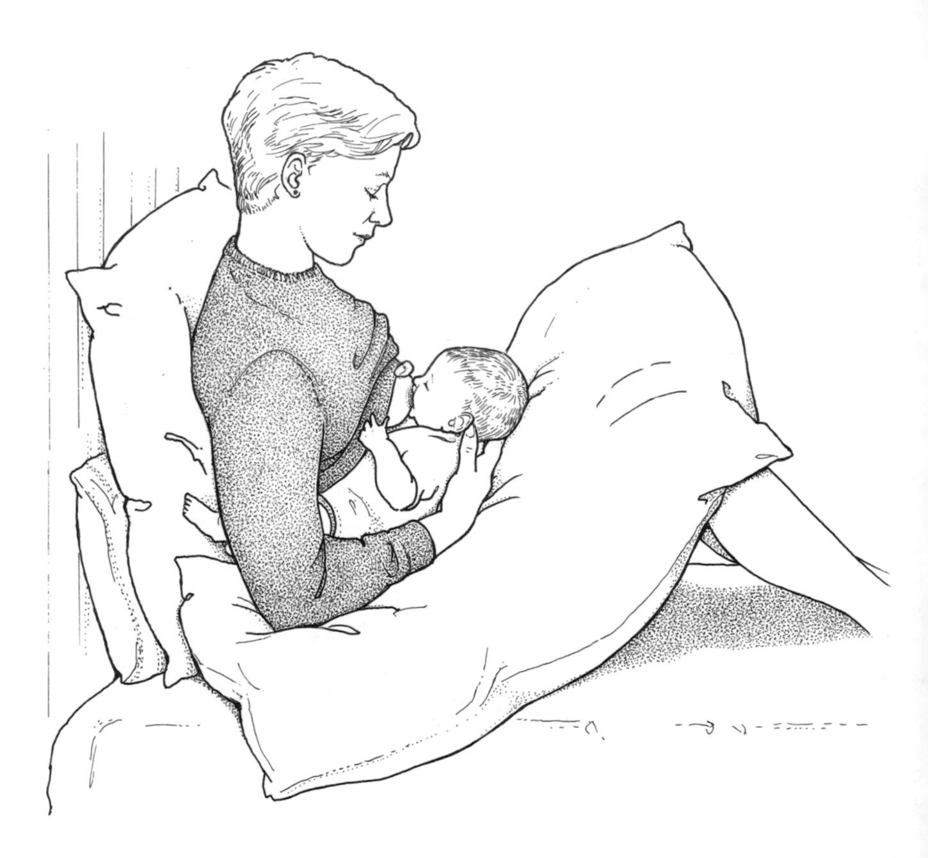

C-HOLD

This is best for moms with large breasts. Place your palm under your breast, with the edge of your hand as close to your chest as possible. (It's OK if your hand isn't touching your chest wall—it's more important to support your breast.) Form the letter C with your hand. Keep your fingers away from the areola, so your fingers don't interfere with the baby's latch. Bring the baby to your nipple, and make sure he gets a big mouthful of nipple. Support your breast lightly (let the breast rest on your hand, rather than gripping it) as the baby nurses.

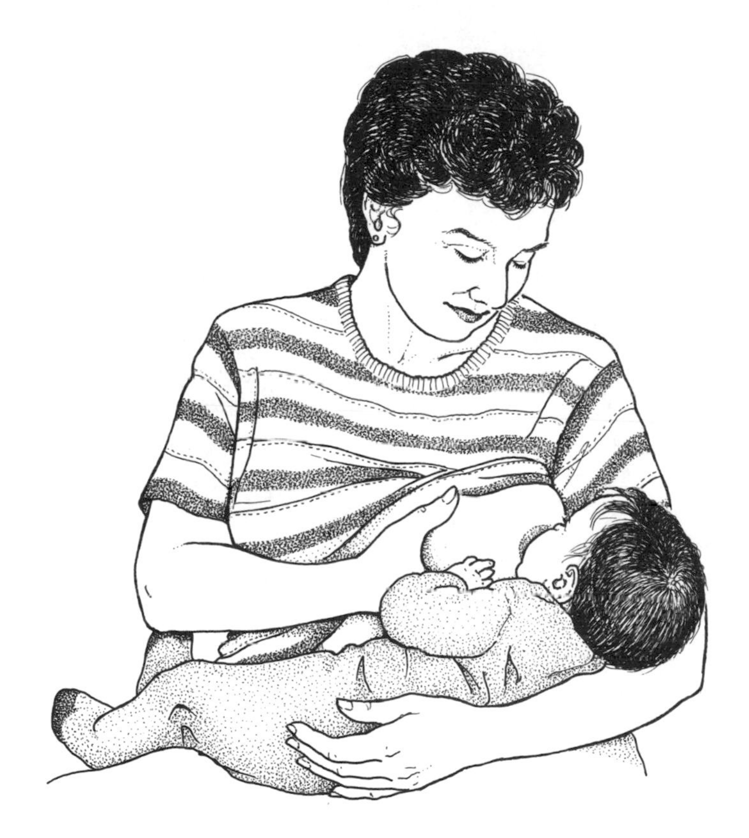

CRADLE HOLD

Cuddle the baby on her side, facing you, belly-to-belly. Rest her head in the crook of your elbow, with your forearm and palm supporting her back and bottom. Bring her head up level with your nipple. Use a pillow to support your elbow and forearm. (A nursing pillow or Boppy is ideal for this position.)

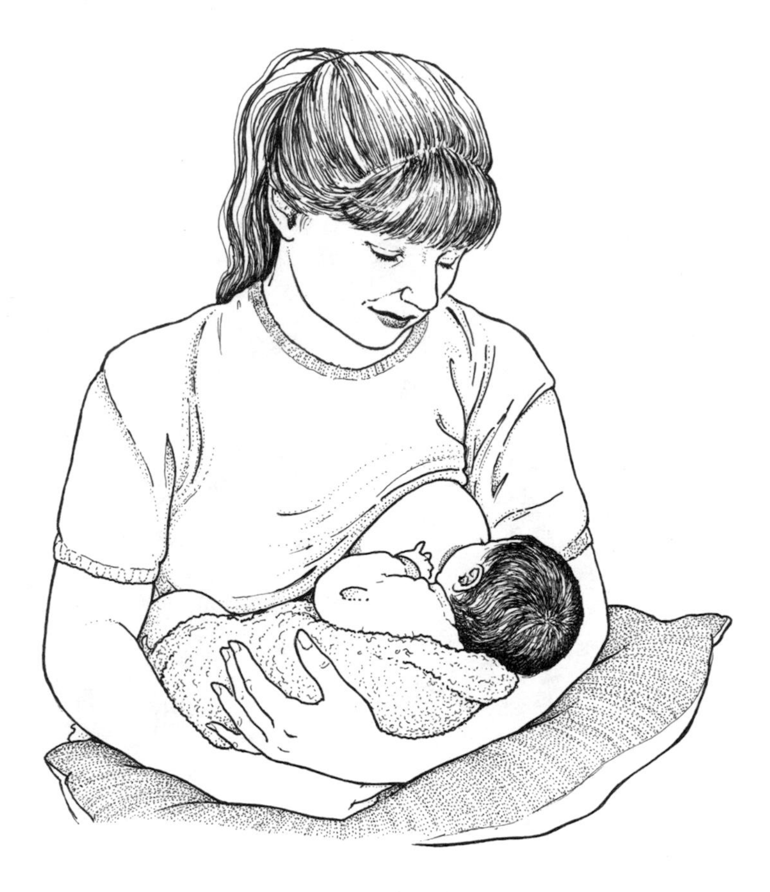

CROSSOVER (REVERSE CRADLE) HOLD

Hold the baby in your right arm, with your hand supporting the baby's head at your left breast. This hold is awkward at first, but it gives you more control, especially if your baby is wiggly or if she only briefly opens her mouth wide enough to latch on.

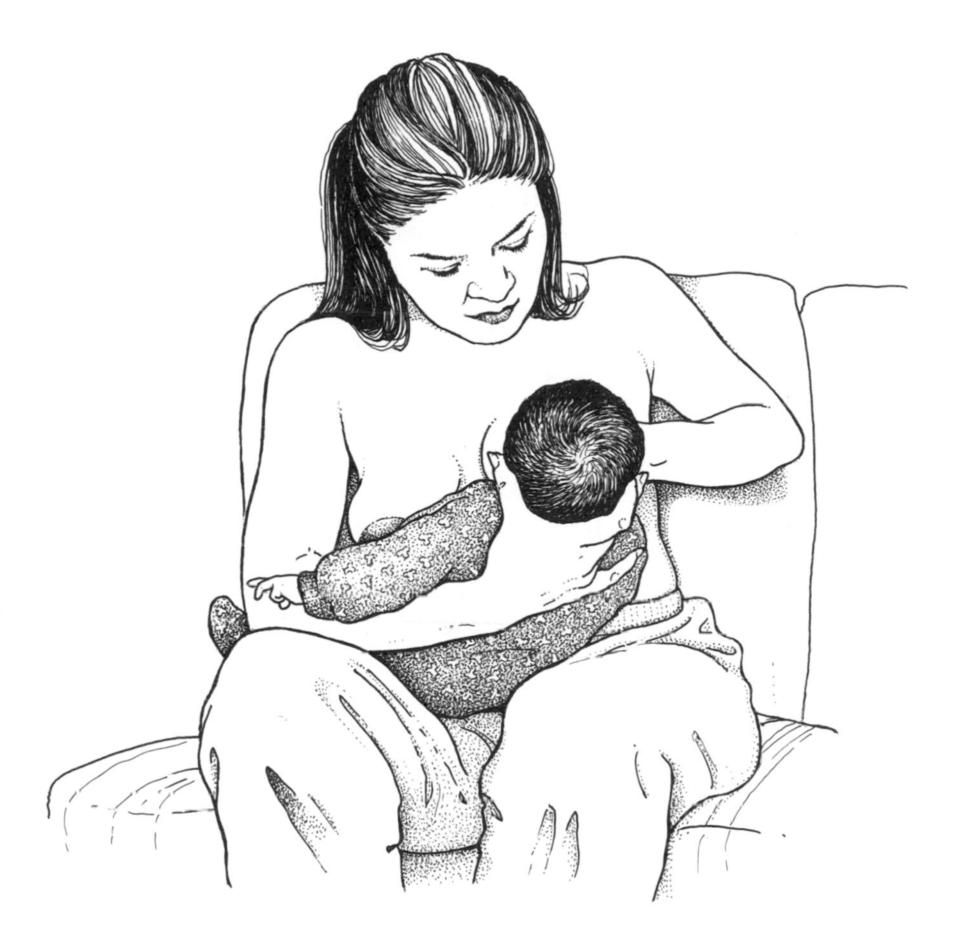

FOOTBALL HOLD

In this position, the baby is tucked under your arm, the way a pro football player carries the ball when he's running for a touchdown. It gives you better control of your baby's head as she latches on.

Hold the baby's head in your hand, facing your breast. Support his back and spine with your forearm and elbow—sort of the opposite of the cradle hold position. He should be tucked against your body with his feet and legs under your armpit.

Use a lot of pillows to bring the baby to *your* level. Resist the temptation to lower your breast to the baby—add more pillows instead. Your back should be supported with lots of pillows, too. Reclining chairs or sofas are better than rockers or chairs with high arms, which interfere with positioning and can be too narrow.

This hold is especially helpful for moms who are recovering from a c-section and for those with large breasts or whose babies are squirmy or arch their backs, or if they're fighting thrush or a breast inflammation or infection.

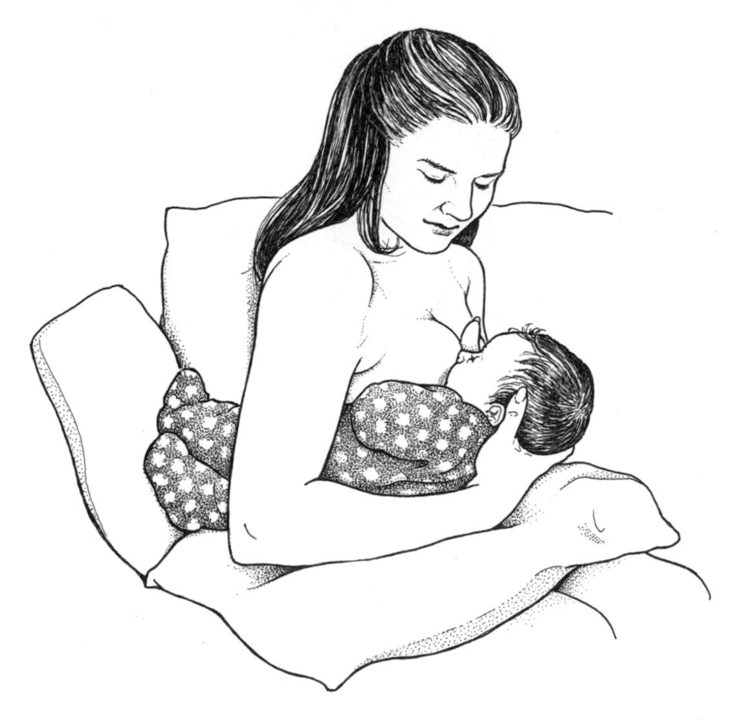

LYING DOWN

Family bed. You and the baby lie on your sides, facing each other. Use pillows behind your back and knees for support and comfort, and a pillow behind the baby's back to prevent her from rolling over. You can also cradle her in your arm, with her back along your forearm and your palm against her skull.

This position is ideal when you're having a nursing holiday, or if you have a family bed to facilitate nighttime nursing.

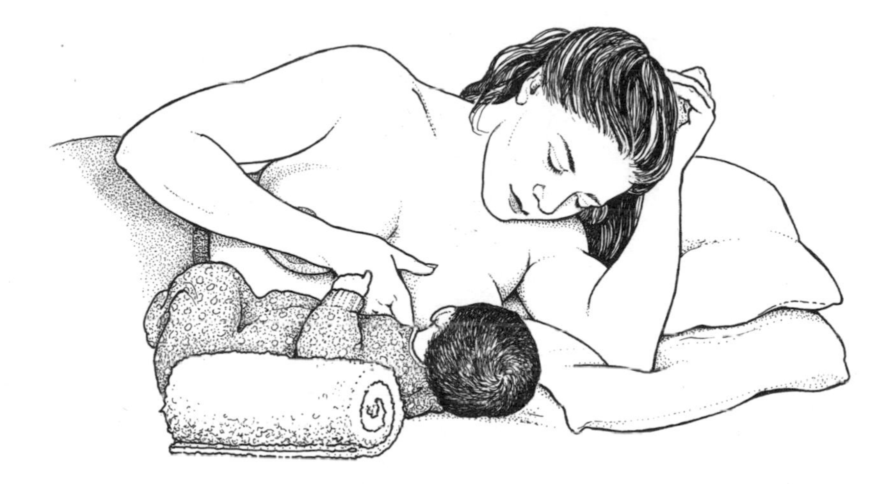

UPSIDE DOWN

Best for older babies with some head and neck control, and good for overactive letdown at any age. Lying flat on your back, latch the baby onto your breast, holding the baby at an angle to your body. He will be halfway on your chest, with his bottom and legs trailing into the air or onto the bed.

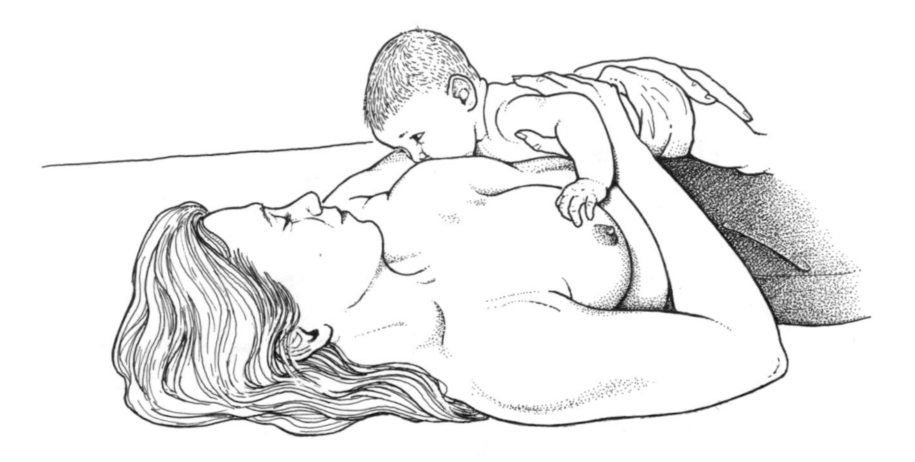

TROUBLESHOOTING

Problem: Baby has trouble staying latched on because of heavy or droopy breasts.

Solution: Hold your breast for him, or use a fabric sling, during the feeding.

Problem: Baby wants to nurse only in cross-cradle position.

Solution: Latch her on with the cross-cradle, and switch to the regular cradle hold in mid-feed. (Very small babies, and babies who have trouble staying latched on, may need the extra support of the cross-cradle hold until they're bigger and more adept at nursing.)

Problem: Nursing with mastitis.

Solution: Lie down on the affected side. Lay your baby down

on her side, with her head pointing down toward your feet, so she can nurse on the infected breast. Her lower lip should be over the plugged/engorged/inflamed area—that's where her suck reflex is strongest. Repeat with every feed until the mastitis clears up. If you don't nurse on the other breast, you must pump it to avoid becoming engorged.

Problem: Nursing out a plugged duct.

Solution: Two positions can help your baby clear a plugged duct.

- Seated: Hold the baby at a 35- to 45-degree angle by sitting on a couple of firm pillows or a cushion (robbed from the unused part of your sofa). Position the baby in the football hold, with her bottom resting next to the cushion, below you, at an angle.
- Lying down: Lie beside the baby, belly-to-belly, with the baby's head and shoulders on a separate pillow, so she can reach your upper breast easily. If you have to lean down so she can get at your breast, rearrange her pillow so that neither you nor the baby is straining. A nursing pillow can be especially helpful.

Problem: Nursing on only one breast per feeding.

Solution: As long as the baby empties your breast, and you offer the other side for the next feeding, this isn't something to worry about.

Problem: Baby goes from taking 15 minutes per breast at each feed to 3–5 minutes apiece.

Solution: If the baby is gaining weight appropriately, and producing enough wet and poopy diapers, how long she nurses is irrelevant. Many babies become efficient nursers as they get older.

WHAT TO AVOID

- Pushing your breast across your body
- Chasing the baby with your breast
- Flapping your breast up and down
- Holding your breast in a scissor grip
- Failing to support your breast

- Twisting your body toward the baby instead of slightly away
- Aiming the nipple at the dead center of the baby's mouth, instead of asymmetrically
- Pulling hard on the baby's chin to force open the mouth
- Flexing the baby's head and neck as you bring the baby to your breast
- Bringing your breast to the baby's mouth, instead of bringing the baby to your breast
- Moving the baby onto the breast before her mouth is yawning open
- Failing to move the baby onto the breast quickly enough when she opens her mouth wide
- Allowing your baby's nose to touch the breast before her chin touches it
- Pressing the breast away from the baby's nose

See also Latching On, About; Nipples, Sore, About

Postpartum Thyroiditis

See Thyroid Scans

Prefers One Breast

Q: My 5-day-old son latches onto my right breast more readily than the left. So my left side becomes engorged and sore, and so hard that even when I try to get him to latch onto that side, he can't. Now he refuses to nurse on the left side at all. What should I do?

A: A lot of babies prefer one breast over the other—usually there's a preference for the breast that has the more abundant supply—so this is a common problem.

Have you tried expressing milk on the left breast before attempting to latch on the baby? That will make it a little easier for him to get a grip on your nipple. Using breast compression on the less preferred breast will help speed up the flow of milk while he's nursing. Most babies like a fast flow of milk. Varying the position you normally use may help, too—try the football hold if you usually use the cradle, or experiment with other positions that could make it easier for him to latch on.

Here's one way to get him to nurse on the left side: Express a little milk, leave some on your nipple, and start him on your left side when he's hungry. He may fuss and cry at first, but if you're persistent, he'll latch on and suckle for a few minutes before starting to fret. Let him nurse on the right breast for a few minutes, and then switch him back to the left. Eventually, he'll be nursing at least a bit on the left side, though it may take a couple of weeks. He may continue to prefer the right breast—it's not unusual for babies to like nursing on one side more than the other.

To relieve the engorgement and maintain your supply, buy or rent a good breast pump and pump the left side. Try holding your son in different positions. It's entirely possible to feed your son adequately from one breast, but it's best to have him nurse from both. (Then, if you get mastitis, you still have a back-up breast.) So be persistent about offering him your left breast.

See also Nipples, Inverted; Positions, About

Pregnancy and Changes in Breast Milk

Q: I just found out that I'm pregnant again, and I'm still nursing my 8-month-old. I heard that hormonal changes associated with pregnancy can alter breast milk. How?

A: Pregnancy affects each mother's milk supply differently. Sometimes, the milk supply dries up almost immediately. Often, the flavor of breast milk starts to change around the 4th or 5th month of pregnancy. Some babies keep nursing, but many self-wean because they don't like the new taste. You will need to supplement as your milk supply drops. As you draw closer to your due date the milk will shift into colostrum to provide antibodies to the new baby.

If your first child is still interested in nursing, and you're will-

ing to juggle nursing a baby and a toddler, the task is formidable but achievable. (And with two babies 17 months apart, tandem nursing would be the least of your problems.) Good luck!
See also Supply Problems, About; Tandem Nursing

Pregnancy and Nursing

Q: I'm nursing a 12-month-old, and I've just learned that I'm pregnant. I'd like to let my son self-wean, but he's still an avid nurser. What's it like to continue nursing throughout a pregnancy? Do I need extra nutrition? Will I be more tired than usual? I want to make a decision that will benefit both my son and the growing baby.

A: You can continue nursing throughout your pregnancy. It's possible your son will self-wean; during pregnancy, hormonal shifts affect the taste of your milk, and some babies don't like the change. Those who self-wean usually stop during the fourth or fifth month of the mother's pregnancy. (In a La Leche League study of 503 mothers, about 69 percent weaned when they were pregnant again.)

One benefit of continuing to nurse throughout pregnancy: It forces your (increasingly active) child to sit down for a few minutes!

You'll have to make some adjustments if your child keeps nursing. Your nipples will be more sensitive, and nursing may be painful. Use relaxation techniques, like Lamaze breathing, to get past the pain, which can be pretty toe-curling.

You'll also need to drink a lot of water—at least 8 ounces every 2 or 3 hours—and get enough protein. Remember that breastfeeding exclusively can burn up an extra 500 calories a day (the total drops as you supplement with other foods), and pregnancy means adding another 200 to 300 calories a day. Managing to meet those requirements may be tough at first, especially if you have morning sickness. If you can't tolerate fruits, veggies, and complex carbohydrates, consider checking out athletic energy bars and gels, sold in some supermarkets and most outdoors and sports stores. They're designed to be digested easily, and they may be one solution for boosting calories without upsetting a sensitive stomach.

Pregnancy and Sensitive Nipples

Q: I'd like to continue nursing at least through the early part of my pregnancy, but my nipples are so hypersensitive that breastfeeding is painful. How can I deal with this?

A: One study of women who continued to breastfeed after they were pregnant found that nearly three fourths of them reported nipple pain or discomfort. During pregnancy, your breasts are very tender, and nursing can exacerbate that.

If you're determined to continue nursing, try varying nursing positions. Explain to your baby that your breasts have "little owies" and that she needs to nurse very gently. You may be able to mitigate some of the pain by hand-expressing a little milk before the baby latches on.

As your pregnancy proceeds, your milk production will drop as your breasts replace the milk with colostrum. This is normal.

It's also not unusual to feel edgy or restless while you're nursing, partly because of your extrasensitive skin and partly in response to the uterine contractions that occur while you are nursing.

Pregnancy Test, Accuracy of While Nursing

Q: Does a home pregnancy test still work if you're breastfeeding heavily?

A: A home pregnancy test measures a human growth hormone that is present only when you are pregnant. It is unaffected by lactation.

Premature Baby, Encouraging to Nurse

Q: My daughter was born at 35 weeks, and I've been pumping for her. I'm worried about my milk production—it seems low, even though the neonatologist says the baby's gaining well.

A: Trust the neonatologist: If your daughter is gaining appropriately, your milk production is fine. It may seem insufficient, because you're still producing milk specifically for a premature baby. Tell your neonatologist that you want to breastfeed as soon as your baby's sucking reflex is mature, and ask for a lactation consultant experienced in working with preemies.

See also Lactation Consultant; Nipple Confusion; Pumping, About; Tube Feeding Lactation Aid

Prenatal Vitamins

Q: Is it true that I should continue to take prenatal vitamins while I'm breastfeeding our new baby? I was planning to go back to my old multivitamin supplement; the prenatals make me nauseated.

A: Taking vitamins while you're breastfeeding is a good way to make sure that you're getting all the essential vitamins and minerals your body needs. Prenatal vitamins pack a powerful punch. Many obstetricians encourage new moms to take prenatal vitamins for at least a month post partum, more or less as a precautionary measure, because childbirth takes such a toll on your body. But after that, a regular multivitamin is fine.

Before then, if you customarily take other vitamin supplements, including iron, eliminate those while you're taking the prenatal vitamins. Prenatal vitamins contain more iron than everyday vitamins, and even the extra iron in prenatal vitamins can cause fussy or colicky behavior in a breastfed baby.

If you suspect you're anemic, ask your doctor to test your hematocrit levels once a month or so. Most moms don't need extra iron if they're also taking prenatal vitamins. If you don't want to take a prenatal vitamin, a good multivitamin usually can handle your daily needs.

See also Pulling on Nipple

Productivity: More in One Breast

Q: I seem to have more milk in my left breast than in my right, and my son prefers the left breast. When I double-pump, I only get a couple of ounces from the right breast, while milk from the left one jets out and produces twice as much. Is this normal?

A: It's normal, and it's common. Most nursing moms notice that one breast typically produces more than the other. If your baby is gaining weight and developing on target, it's not something to worry about. You may be able to increase the supply on the low-productivity breast by encouraging your baby to nurse first on that side and by using breast compression as she nurses. (*See* Breast Compression.) But often babies have a definite breast preference—and, not surprisingly, the breast they like better is the one that produces more milk.

Public, Nursing in

See Breastfeeding in Public, About

Pulling on Nipple

Q: My son is gaining weight well—he's gone from 7 pounds at birth to 15 pounds at 11 weeks—but he pulls my nipple so hard when he nurses that I'm getting sore. I know he's not pulling to get milk. (Once I sprayed my husband when he was walking by as my son unlatched.) How can I get him to stop pulling?

A: Guess what: Your overactive letdown—evidenced by your spraying milk—may be the problem. Does your son seem to "glug" as he nurses? Does he tend to pull at the start of a feed? If he does, the pulling is probably due to an overactive letdown. He may be pulling away from the milk spraying into his mouth, attempting to control the flow.

Try expressing some milk before nursing, until the milk stops spraying, and then latch him on.

Other techniques:

- Nurse from one breast only in a 2- to 4-hour time period.

- Nurse lying down.
- Ask a physician specializing in lactation issues about giving your baby simethicone drops.

It's also possible that your son is sensitive to something in your diet. Does he seem unhappy when he's nursing? Pull off, and toss his head? Does he seem cranky after a feed? Dairy is the usual suspect when a baby is sensitive to something in a mother's diet. (*See* Allergies (Baby's), About.)

Another possibility: overdosing on iron. Do you take iron supplements? Too much iron can make a baby's stomach rebellious. Prenatal vitamins, or even regular multivitamins, can contain enough iron to affect a baby's stomach.

See also Colic; Allergies, Dairy; Prenatal Vitamins

Pumping, About

EVALUATING BREAST PUMPS

There are four kinds of pumps: hospital-grade, professional-grade, small electric, and manual. Rental pumps are usually hospital- or professional-grade. If you buy a pump, look first at what a couple of local rental companies offer. A good rule of thumb is to avoid buying a pump that a rental company won't carry. If money is an issue, buy a good secondhand pump instead of a cheap new one. Whether you rent or buy, you must use a new attachment kit—the part that contains breast flanges, tubing, collection bottles, and shields. Never use secondhand attachment kits: It's impossible to sterilize them completely.

Hospital-grade pumps are extremely expensive to own—they cost between $800 and $2,000. However, they're efficient and durable, and invaluable to a mom who pumps a lot, e.g., a mom who has a premature or ill baby, or one who is determined to use breast milk even if she's physically unable to nurse. (In a case like that, insurance may cover the rental costs of a hospital-grade pump.) Hospital-grade pumps can be used for double- or single-pumping.

Among the best hospital-grade pumps are these:

- Medela Classic: widely used in hospitals. Advantages: strong, tough, efficient. Downside: very heavy (20 pounds) and expensive.
- Medela Lactina Select: carried by most pump rental businesses. Advantages: strong, durable, light, with a dial that adjusts for speed and suction level, and an insulated area for chilling milk. Downside: cost.

Professional-grade pumps are almost as efficient as hospital-grade pumps. Because they're designed for individual use, they lack a hospital-grade filtering system. Like hospital pumps, the attachments allow double- or single-pumping. Professional-grade pumps are intended for daily use and will last 2 years or more.

Among the best professional-grade pumps are these:

- Medela Pump in Style. Advantages: adjustable speed and suction, double-pumping option, light weight, attache-style shoulder bag that contains kit parts and has an insulated storage area for milk. Disadvantage: expensive.
- Purely Yours (Ameda-Egnell). Advantages: adjustable speed and suction, less expensive and lighter than Pump in Style. Disadvantages: more affordable than Pump in Style, but still expensive.

Small electric pumps are designed for users who pump infrequently—for a parent's night out, or a short trip away from home. At about $100, they're more affordable than professional-grade pumps, but also less durable and often noisy.

One warning about electric pumps: Avoid those made by companies that also sell formula; their pumps almost invariably are uncomfortable, inefficient, and flimsy.

Two good small electric pumps are these:

- Medela Mini-Electric. Advantages: hand-held, with battery back-up, auto-cycle, effective for short-term use, with manual pump option. In its price category (about $60), probably the best affordable pump. Disadvantage: louder than an electric razor.

- Nurture III. Advantages: double-pumping option, with some advantages of a professional-grade pump. Disadvantage: doesn't auto-cycle, and releasing suction requires you to fiddle with the collection bottles.

Manual pumps vary in price and quality. If your milk supply is just coming in, a manual pump is far less efficient and effective than an electric pump, and much more difficult to use. Again, don't bother with manual pumps made by companies that sell formula or bottles. The big exception: Avent, whose pumps are enormously popular with nursing moms. Three commendable manual pumps are these:

- Avent Isis. Advantage: affordable (about $50), easy to use, gentle and effective with petal-style suction that massages the nipples. Many moms compare the Isis favorably to electric pumps. Disadvantage: lots of parts to assemble.
- Egnell One-hand Breast pump. About $40, but some hospitals give it away free. Advantage: very comfortable. Disadvantage: the squeeze-action operation is a little tough to master.
- Medela SpringExpress. About $30. Advantages: effective, and your biceps will look terrific—this pump uses your large arm muscles to operate a plunger. Disadvantage: your biceps will protest at first, and it's not as easy to use as other manual pumps.

Many electric pumps have battery packs (about $160 or so apiece, or $15 or so in monthly rental charges), so you can use them when there's no outlet nearby. (Possible downside: Battery packs are bulky, and often there's no extra space for them in pump carrying cases or bags.) Some pumps have converters; you can run the Pump in Style and the Purely Yours on the voltage from a car's cigarette lighter plug. (Must we add that it's not a good idea to do this when you are driving?)

Most breast pumps require you to clasp the breast flanges against your breasts. Some pumps will stop if you break the suction. If you need your hands for other tasks, you can try the

Hands-Free Attachment kit, which basically holds the shields to your breasts with modified rubber bands. Medela makes a hands-free pumping bra. (Warning: Avoid multitasking yourself to death. Pumping offers a rare chance for a pause during an especially hectic time of life.)

PUMPING AT HOME

If you're pumping at home and are having trouble coaxing much milk from your breasts when you pump, try pumping on one side when the baby nurses on the other. Your suckling baby will stimulate even the unused breast, and you'll get more milk than if you're using the pump alone. Use a pillow on your lap to support the baby, and keep a hand free for holding the pump's breast cup in place.

Some women pump before they nurse, especially if they have an overactive letdown and an abundant milk supply; others pump afterward.

PUMPING AT WORK

If you're pumping at work, ask the company's human resource staff about being able to use an empty office for pumping.

Sometimes, the only place available to pump is a restroom. This is not hygienic, and it should only be used as a last resort. If there is nothing but a counter and stalls, your best bet is to use the counter to set up the pump. (If there's no outlet, bring a long orange power cord and plug it into the nearest outlet.)

If the counter won't work, you can use the handicapped-access stall, which is large enough to accommodate an extra chair. It's hardly ideal—you'll have to be scrupulous about washing your hands and using paper towels to open, close, and latch the stall door, and you should check with any staffer whose disability requires using this stall.

If your office has a refrigerator, use it to store bags of expressed milk during the day. Get a metal box and label it with your baby's name and yours, using indelible ink. Keep the bags of milk in the box, and keep it against the back wall, where it's coldest. Take the box of bags home every day. (True story: An overzealous co-worker once threw out a week's worth of frozen, expressed milk, assuming the little plastic bags were abandoned. He is lucky to still be alive.)

HOW MUCH TO PUMP

Your baby consumes roughly 2.5 to 3 ounces (75 to 90 grams) of expressed milk per pound of body weight each day. When you calculate how much milk to leave with your baby's caregiver, divide the total amount of milk consumed daily and divide it by the number of times he nurses in 24 hours. Err on the safe side by adding an ounce or so more when you first leave your baby with someone else, in case you run late or the baby is especially hungry.

See also Pumping: Estimating the Baby's Needs

TRANSPORTING EXPRESSED MILK

For short commutes (less than 20 minutes), store the small bags of expressed milk in a large sealed baggie or a small insulated bag, with a layer of ice, a freezer cold pack, or a bag of frozen peas to keep the milk cool.

For longer commutes and flights, use a small Styrofoam cooler (small enough to stash under an airline seat). Line the bottom of the cooler with an old towel (to absorb anything that melts or spills), and put bags of expressed milk on top of the towel (one layer, if the milk is not frozen; if the milk is frozen, you can stack the bags like bricks). Over this, put a couple of layers of newspaper. Cover the newspaper with chunks of dry ice (available at ice-cream specialty stores). If you're flying, call the airline before you buy the dry ice. If the carrier won't allow dry ice on board, several layers of wadded newspaper will keep frozen milk cold enough to reach your destination.

Seal the cooler with plastic packing tape or duct tape. This will keep the milk frozen solid as a rock for at least 8 hours. Carry the cooler on board if you're flying: Styrofoam coolers may crack and break when the luggage shifts inside the plane. (You can also ship milk overnight by mail or United Parcel Service, and it will stay frozen if you pack it in a box, not a Styrofoam cooler.)

PUMPING TIPS

- If you have trouble letting down enough milk at first, jump-start things by expressing some milk by hand.
- It will take a few days before you see a measurable increase in supply. Don't give up because you're discouraged by seeing what seems like little or no increase.
- If your nipples are tender, use lubricant, like a lanolin-based ointment, on them before you start pumping.
- Don't be surprised if you pump only an ounce (or less) at first. Pumps are less efficient than babies at getting milk from your breasts, and until you get used to the sensation of the pump's suction, you may be unable to relax enough for your letdown to really kick in.
- When you're away from the baby, pump at the times you'd normally nurse.
- When your baby is nursing frequently, try pumping afterward. You'll produce more milk when you pump, and she'll also get more milk when she nurses.
- It's not unusual for the productive breast to be slightly larger than the other one.
- Experiment with the pressure and speed. Too much pressure can cause red, sore nipples—and you won't get more milk, anyway.
- Small heat-sealers, like the Eurosealer, are enormously helpful for storing expressed milk in bags. The milk is sealed airtight, and the bags are virtually spillproof. A small heat-sealer runs on two AA batteries (though some are electric) and is available at kitchen specialty stores and department stores for less than $20.
- If you have trouble relaxing when you begin pumping, stash a picture of your baby in your pump's carrying

case. Prop the photo where you can see it as you pump. Some moms say their productivity increases by nearly half.

- Listen to a favorite tape while you pump. Try soothing instrumental music or a calming nature tape. A 1989 University of New Mexico study quoted in the American Academy of Pediatrics magazine reported that mothers who pumped or expressed milk improved their production by 63 percent after listening to a 20-minute audio cassette tape based on relaxation and visual imagery techniques. The same study found that anxiety, fatigue, and emotional stress had a powerful and negative effect on lactation and milk production.
- Save some time by using disposable bottle bags to line your pump bottles. You can use disposable bags sold alongside formula in supermarkets, or bags made specifically for pumps (Mother's Milk and Medela's CSF are two good brands). You can put the bags directly into the freezer.
- Start out pumping once every 2-1/2 hours when you're away from the baby, to stimulate milk supply. After a month, skip the first pumping session, and see how much milk you get from the second session. Some moms find that they can get more from pumping only once or twice a day than from several pumping sessions.
- Wash, and separate, the three parts of pump components each time you pump. If you use your dishwasher, always put the components on the top rack; they may melt on the bottom rack. Milk banks require donor moms to boil the breast shields and inserts for 20 minutes. (If you disinfect by boiling, use a loud timer. It's easy to get so distracted that the pot boils dry, melting the pump parts.)
- Flanges and filters melt and get lost in dishwashers. You can special-order baskets from Medela and other pump companies. For an inexpensive alternative, use two open-weave plastic strawberry baskets, put the inserts

inside, and fasten the baskets with twist-ties. The parts will last longer if you remove them before the dishwasher goes into the drying cycle.

- If you don't have time to disinfect the parts once a week, buy an extra set. This is especially handy if you pump full time, or pump at work.
- If you pump at work, wear tops that can be pulled free of a skirt or pants, or a shirtwaist dress. Turtlenecks, pullover dresses, back-zipped dresses or tops, and jumpers are logistically troublesome and leave you more exposed if someone inadvertently interrupts a pumping session.
- Lean forward when you pump. It can improve your milk flow.
- Massage your breast as you pump. That helps the milk flow, too.
- Pump one breast while you nurse. It will improve your overall milk supply as well as your back-up stock.
- Some pumps have adapters—handy if you have one type at home and another at work or when you're traveling. Avent's adapter (about $10) makes it possible to use Medela and other pumps while pumping directly into your Avent bottles. It saves a lot of pouring.

STORING AND USING EXPRESSED MILK

- Label bags by date. This reminds you and other caregivers to use older stock first.
- Fresh expressed milk can be stored in the refrigerator for 8 days, according to a 1996 study.
- Unrefrigerated expressed milk will keep at room temperature for 15 hours before spoiling.
- Chill expressed milk before you freeze it, instead of putting it into the freezer warm.
- If you're interrupted while you're pumping, you can put the pump's bottles into the refrigerator, and—after washing your hands well—take them back out later to pump more milk. This is recommended only if you're in a

pinch, not on a regular basis.

- Store frozen breast milk in bags containing 2 to 3 ounces apiece, in the middle and back of the freezer. If you use a frost-free freezer, do not put milk next to the freezer walls.
- Never store frozen breast milk in the freezer door. Opening and closing the door will generate enough heat to thaw the milk enough to spoil it.
- About 20 to 30 ounces of frozen expressed milk will fit in one large (half-gallon) Ziploc freezer bag.
- Always mark the date on the bag (or bottle) of freshly expressed milk. A dry-erase marker works on most plastic bottles. Be sure to also note any medication you've taken. Some moms even note what they ate, especially if their last meal was something unusual.
- Thaw frozen milk in warm water. Never use a microwave to thaw or warm expressed milk.
- Frozen breast milk can be thawed in the refrigerator but must be used within 24 hours.
- If expressed milk looks curdled, it's probably soured, even if it's odorless. Toss it.
- It's OK to mix formula with expressed breast milk, although the lactoferrin protein in the breast milk binds to the iron in the formula, decreasing the iron in both. The same thing happens in a baby's digestive system if you don't allow 20 to 30 minutes between feeding a baby expressed breast milk and formula, or iron-enriched baby cereal and breast milk.
- If a baby hasn't finished a bottle of expressed milk, you can use it within the next 24 hours, but after that, toss it out.
- Fresh expressed milk can be added to expressed milk pumped earlier that day, and then frozen.
- Frozen expressed milk can be stored near the back (the coldest part) of a regular freezer for 3 to 6 months, and in a deep-freeze for 6 months.

- Avoid using cheap bags. They split easily. To keep bags in shape, put each bag inside a paper cup, and then freeze.

TROUBLESHOOTING

- Expressed milk is thick and clumping: Could be a sign of mastitis, especially if you've had a history of breast inflammations, infections, or previous bouts of mastitis. There may be bacteria in your milk. See a doctor immediately; if it is mastitis, you need to go on antibiotics. In any case, the milk should be cultured in a laboratory, and you should be assessed for symptoms that indicate other problems. (*See also* Clumping Milk.)
- Expressed milk separates in two layers: This is normal. Milk that isn't homogenized does separate into cream and thin milk. It is not spoiled unless it smells bad or looks curdled.
- Curdled-looking expressed milk: Small clots float in milk, odd smell and/or taste. It's curdled. Dump it.
- Frozen milk is chalky, may smell odd (but not sour) when thawed: Did you chill the milk before freezing it? Warm breast milk that goes straight to the freezer can assume a chalky texture and scent. It's OK to use, as long as your baby doesn't mind.
- Blood in expressed milk: Could be a sign of inflammation or infection. See a doctor immediately, in case you need antibiotics.
- Soapy odor in frozen milk: Caused by an enzyme in breast milk that breaks down during the freezing process, causing the milk to take on a different odor. If the baby doesn't mind the taste or smell, don't worry. It should taste like regular breast milk—if it tastes off, it's sour and should be tossed.

Pumping, and Decreasing Milk Supply

Q: My 10-month-old still nurses six or seven times a day, and I've been pumping to get a bit extra to store in the freezer. Lately, I've been able to pump only 4 ounces a day in two pumping sessions. I used to be able to pump 4 to 6 ounces at a time. Now I'm lucky to get 2 ounces at each session. Isn't increased demand supposed to lead to increased supply?

A: Most moms who pump run into this problem. The reason: Your body responds better to a baby than to a breast pump. Usually, babies are much more efficient than breast pumps at eliciting milk. They only get more efficient as they get older (the babies, not the pumps).

Theoretically, increased demand leads to increased supply. But the pump doesn't demand as much of your breasts as the baby does, so your breasts don't produce as much milk when you pump.

At 10 months, your baby is probably eating some solids, and your breasts just aren't making as much milk as they did when he depended exclusively on breast milk.

Pumping: Estimating the Baby's Needs

Q: Is there a way to calculate how much expressed milk to give our baby's day care provider? We're still struggling to get the baby to take a bottle, so it's hard to get a reliable take on how much she's eating.

A: The general guideline for calculating a baby's total daily needs is 150 to 180 milliliters, or 5 to 6 ounces, of breast milk or formula per kilo of body weight. (One kilo is 2.2 pounds.)

Divide this amount by the number of times she nurses each day to determine approximately how much she'll take at a time. For example, if an 11-pound (5-kilogram) baby feeds seven times a day, she needs about 3-1/2 ounces (110 milliliters) per feeding. You might want to add an ounce or so more, and let her decide how much she wants. After about a week, you'll get a better idea of her needs.

This is a guideline, not a rigid formula. Play it safe: Send a couple ounces more milk than you think she needs, until you and the day care provider figure out the right amount. To avoid wasting expressed milk, freeze your pumped milk in 2-ounce bags.

Remember that your baby's eating patterns will change during growth spurts and milestones, like teething and learning to roll over, sit up, and crawl. If she's nursing more at home, send a little extra to day care. See if your provider is willing to store a few ounces of extra milk in her freezer for you. Then she'll have enough for a back-up bottle when your baby's appetite increases unexpectedly.

See also Pumping, About

Pumping During Pregnancy

Q: If I start pumping before I'm due, will that help my milk come in? I've heard that it can prevent becoming engorged.

A: Pumping before your due date is a bad idea. It can stimulate uterine contractions, causing premature labor.

See Pumping, About

Pumping, Tapering Off

Q: With a tight schedule, I'm proud that I've managed to pump two or three times a day for 6 months, but now I'm ready to stop. How, exactly, do I go about weaning my breasts from the pump? I don't want to be miserable. Also, I want to continue nursing at home on weekends and in the mornings and evenings. Will my supply keep up?

A: Congratulations for pumping so long. If you're like most moms who pump, you may have noticed that you're getting less and less from pumping as time passes. Start by pumping a little less each day for 3 or 4 days. Then skip a pumping session once every 3 to 5 days. If you feel uncomfortably engorged, then you probably are trying to wean too fast. You may find as you cut back on the number of times you pump each day that you actually collect more milk by the day's end.

To taper off the last pumping session, pump 1 day, skip the next, and pump the day after that. Then go 2 days without pumping.

Expect to be a little engorged, especially if you continue nursing at home. (You'll be ready to nurse by the time you walk in the door!) But you should feel full, not tight as a tick.

There's no reason to stop nursing at home just because you're not pumping at work. Your supply should keep up with your baby's demand at this point.

Pumps, Electric

Q: Everyone tells me that I *must* use an electric pump if I'm working. They say that manual pumps are good only for reducing engorgement, not for stockpiling expressed milk or for maintaining your supply. I've done pretty well so far with my Avent Isis, but I'm not back at work yet. Do I need an electric pump?

A: Not necessarily. Women vary quite a bit in terms of how easily, and how much, they can pump. If you're having success with a manual pump, why not take it to work and see how it goes? You can always rent an electric pump later. Isis is a manual pump that is particularly popular with nursing moms. They like it because they can pump anywhere, and it is exceptionally efficient.

There are several options between a manual and a heavy-duty electric pump like Medela's Pump-in-Style (PIS). Some moms are happy with the Medela mini-electric. The two main drawbacks: it's a noisy critter, and the mini-electrics tend to burn out. However, Medela's mini-electric self-cycles and has plenty of power, and it's a lot cheaper than the PIS.

See also Pumping, About

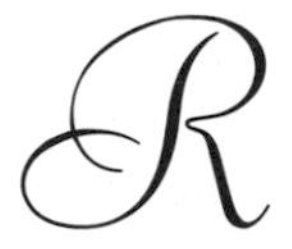

Radial Keratotomy and Breastfeeding

See Vision Correcting Surgery and Breastfeeding

Red Nipples

See Nipples, Sore, About

Red Streak

Q: I've noticed a wiggly red streak, almost like a stretch mark, on my left breast, an inch or so above the nipple. I can still nurse on that breast, but it's becoming tender and hot. What's wrong?

A: The red streak, accompanied by the tenderness, indicates a plugged duct. It could lead to mastitis. See a physician immediately for an accurate diagnosis. If it is an infected duct, your physician probably will prescribe cephalexin, which has little to no effect on your breast milk and acts quickly. (You should be feeling better within 24 to 48 hours; if not, the antibiotic may not be working, and you should return to your physician.)

See also Plugged Ducts, About; Mastitis, About

Reflux, Gastroesophageal

Q: My 12-week-old son was just diagnosed with reflux. I'd like to keep giving him breast milk, but he won't nurse. He's losing weight, and my pediatrician wants me to switch to formula.

A: Get a second opinion. Breastfed babies generally have fewer problems with reflux than formula-fed babies. Gastroesophageal reflux is a complicated medical condition that increasingly is diagnosed in babies. It is a medical problem that can cause feeding problems, because the baby learns to associate eating with pain. Reflux also is one of the most overdiagnosed disorders. Many, if not most, babies experience reflux, but it is not a problem unless the baby has problems gaining weight.

In most cases, gastroesophageal reflux is caused by the baby's immature intestinal tract. In some cases of reflux, babies like your son refuse to nurse because they've learned that eating causes their pain. Teaching them to nurse again takes patience and time.

Some techniques that help:

- Hand-express some milk to jump-start your letdown before latching on the baby.
- Nurse him while he's sleeping.
- Nurse him while you're standing or walking (a sling is helpful).
- Nurse him while you're both sitting in a warm bath; the warm water will help relax you both.
- Keep him upright while nursing (to discourage the milk from coming back up).
- Nurse him in a recliner, or propped by pillows that put you at a 45-degree angle, tummy-to-tummy. Having the baby positioned with his head up makes it more likely that when he burps, it will be air, not milk.
- Nurse or feed your baby more frequently, so the feeds are smaller and more manageable.

Other babies with reflux want to nurse constantly. Breast milk acts as a natural antacid.

A reflux baby who likes to nurse should be nursed on only one breast at a time. He's less likely to overfill his stomach. (Even though your breast seems empty, a lactating breast constantly produces milk.)

Cimetidine (Tagamet) and other drugs can control reflux-related irritation in the stomach or esophagus and discourage vomiting. Other reflux medications, such as cisapride (Propulsid), act by stimulating the gastrointestinal tract's rhythmic movements, so there's less in the stomach to reflux back up the esophagus. Cimetidine (Tagamet) and ranitidine (Zantec) both reduce acid production, which is helpful in relieving the irritation, especially in the lower esophagus, that can result from reflux; both medications also help heal the irritated tissue that, untreated, is increasingly unable to function normally. All medications do have side effects: Propulsid may cause heart arhythmia, especially when taken with certain antibiotics. Ask about side effects before agreeing to a medicine, and alert your pharmacist to which medications your baby is taking before adding another. Make sure your pediatrician keeps you updated about any new information.

Untreated, reflux can lead to other feeding disorders that can threaten your baby's life. About one third of the babies diagnosed with reflux also have apnea. Monitor your baby's breathing when he sleeps. If it's irregular, with gaps of several seconds every 10 minutes, talk to your pediatrician about putting him on a monitor. If there are many long pauses in his breathing—a lapse that lasts up to 30 seconds more than once every half hour, call your pediatrician immediately.

Reflux, or Spit-up?

Q: My 6-week-old daughter spits up almost every time I breastfeed her. The spit-up looks sort of like large-curd cottage cheese. Could this be reflux? If it's spit-up, how much do babies normally spit up?

A: Most babies spit up a little after they eat. One difference between spit-up and vomit: Babies spit up only a teaspoon to a tablespoon; when they vomit, they empty everything in their stomachs—several ounces' worth. Dump a tablespoon of water on the kitchen counter, then a quarter cup of water. There's a significant difference.

Gastroesophageal reflux describes what happens when the stomach's contents are being splashed or pushed backward and up into the esophagus and sometimes out the mouth. When a baby throws up most of what she's eaten after nearly every feeding, and between feedings, she may have gastroesophageal reflux. Even very young babies, like yours, can have reflux. Usually, they outgrow it.

Normal spit-up usually happens within 10 minutes of a feed. Usually, a baby spits up only a few tablespoons' worth. If he's gaining well and is happy, spitting up is not a problem (except when it comes to laundry).

Among the symptoms of pathologic reflux: extreme fussiness—crying inconsolably, screaming, arching (especially while nursing), hiccuping, gagging, choking—during waking periods; spitting up after feedings, and an hour or more afterward; hoarse voice; red throat; congestion; and audible, and sometimes strained, breathing. Weight gain is slow to negligible (reflux babies may be diagnosed with failure to thrive). Some babies with reflux refuse to eat; others want to nurse constantly, despite difficulty swallowing.

Some reflux babies have projectile vomiting. Some babies spit up and reswallow, which can cause the trachea and larynx to swell and cause more breathing difficulties.

Consequences of reflux include frequent ear infections, respiratory problems (wheezing, labored breath, asthma, bronchitis, pneumonia, apnea), failure to thrive, and sleeping disorders. See your doctor first.

There are many simple things that can help correct reflux. For more severe problems, consult a pediatric (not an adult) gastroenterologist.

See also Allergies (Baby's), About; Reflux, Gastroesophageal; Spitting Up

Refusing to Nurse: Fussy Baby

Q: Our 3-month-old daughter gets one bottle of expressed milk or formula during the day but nurses the rest of the time. Lately, she won't nurse. She'll start to suck, and then fuss and refuse my nipple, and then latch on again, repeating the whole cycle. It's not a supply problem: Milk squirts out when she pops off the breast. So what's wrong?

A: Maybe several things. The most likely possibilities are that she's going through a growth spurt or starting to teethe—two milestones that provoke this reaction. It could be a case of nipple confusion, although with just one bottle a day, that's probably unlikely.

See also Growth Spurts, About; Nipple Confusion; Nursing Strike; Overactive Letdown; Teething and Nursing

Refusing to Nurse: Milk Tastes "Bad"

Q: My son was in the hospital for the first 2 weeks of his life because of complications associated with his premature birth. While he was in the hospital, he got a combination of breast milk (from a milk bank because I had trouble pumping) and formula. My supply was down, but I was still producing milk when he came home. He latched on fine, but took one swallow and screamed. He refused to nurse again. Finally I tasted my milk, and it was awful. Can breast milk spoil inside your breasts?

A: No. But different factors can change its taste—a change in your diet, a breast infection, pregnancy, going several days between feeding or pumping sessions. When you're weaning a baby, for example, the breast milk starts to taste salty and unappealing.

It's possible that because you couldn't breastfeed and had trouble pumping, your breasts began reacting as if they were weaning. If pumping is not an option for you, but you're determined to relactate and breastfeed, get help from a lactation consultant.

Relactating

Q: Foolishly, I weaned my baby at 3 weeks. Now, she's 6 weeks old and we haven't found a kind of formula she can tolerate. Have you got any advice on how I can relactate?

A: It's possible to relactate with determination on your part. Contact your local La Leche League (1-800-LA-LECHE) to find a lactation consultant who specializes in mothers with difficult issues. She may suggest using a tube feeding lactation aid, like SNS or Lact-Aid, to stimulate your breasts. You can also ask your doctor about the possibility of taking metaclopramide (Reglan), a prescription drug that facilitates lactation, or try herbal galactagues. (*See* Herbal Remedies and Supplements, About.)

Since you're still in the recent postpartum period, it should be a little easier for you to relactate than it is for a woman with an older baby or an adoptive mother who's never been pregnant. In those cases, it's still possible to lactate—one study reported in *Pediatrics* found that six mothers 10 to 150 days post partum, and one adoptive mother, were able to relactate or induce lactation. Each suckled her infant at regular feeding intervals and also used a supplemental feeding device.

One caveat about relactating: You may still need to supplement. Of the mothers in the study, three were able to supply their infants' complete nutritional needs; the others needed to supplement half or more of their babies' diet.

Relaxing While Nursing

Q: I have a 3-week-old baby. It's always a struggle to breastfeed. The baby and I are both tense. I have a hard time with letdown, and I think if I could relax, it would be easier on us. Can you help?

A: For a short-term fix, ask your obstetrician for a prescription for oxytocin nasal spray. That can prompt an almost immediate letdown. You can use the spray for only a very limited time—less than a week, maximum—but it may help you both through a tough time, and teach you to trust yourselves.

Long term: After she latches on, take deep, long breaths—think yoga, not Lamaze—when you nurse. As you exhale, visualize the milk letting down through your breasts into the baby's mouth. This technique sounds awfully touchy-feely, but you'll be surprised: By the third or fourth breath, you'll feel the letdown.

More tips:

- Before you sit down with the baby, put on some soothing music, and focus on it as you nurse.
- Have your partner rub his knuckles down your spine as you nurse—like giving you a spinal noogie. It can work pretty well.
- Try different nursing positions. Very young babies sometimes find it easier to latch on and nurse when they're lying next to you, or tucked in the football hold.
- Get out of the house. Talk a walk with the baby in the stroller, a sling, or a baby carrier. Stroll through a mall, a museum, or an art gallery if the weather's inclement. Most babies enjoy going for a walk, and the time alone may help both of you bond and relax.
- Arrange for some time alone. New mothers often get "touched out" and overstressed. A couple of hours with a friend, a long soak in the tub, or a haircut can give you some breathing room and peace. If your spouse or a family member can't babysit, see if you can trade time with another mom (mothers with toddlers or older children often enjoy watching a baby for a couple of hours).
- If you're drinking coffee, caffeinated sodas, or teas, switch to decaf and water for a couple of weeks.

See also Positions, About

Respiratory Illness

Q: My 2-month-old son has a respiratory infection, and his pediatrician told me I shouldn't be breastfeeding him. Why on earth not?

A: Your son's pediatrician's information is inaccurate. There's an old myth that milk shouldn't be given to children with respiratory illnesses. The jury's out on whether that's true for dairy products. However, breastfeeding will help your son recover more quickly, and it will comfort him and you.

Rocking Chair vs. Glider

Q: I want to set up my nursing area before my baby is born next month. Should I get a rocker or a glider for the chair? Or would an oversized armchair be better? And is a nursing footrest worth the money it costs?

A: It's a good idea to arrange your nursing station before the baby is born. Some new mothers have enough energy to shop for furniture, but most of us consider a typical postpartum day a success if we manage to shower before sunset. If you do buy a new piece of furniture, hang onto the receipt. If it's uncomfortable for nursing, you probably can exchange it—within reason. When in doubt, protect the upholstery with a sheet or blanket to catch spit-up and other leaks.

Which chair to choose is another one of those your-mileage-may-vary topics. Devotees of gliders vastly prefer them to rocking chairs, and vice versa. Though an oversized armchair is cozy, it's better as a supplemental chair. Babies and toddlers tend to prefer the soothing motion of a chair that rocks or glides.

If you're tempted to buy the kind of chair many hospitals use—a combination easy chair/recliner/rocker—think twice. Some toddlers have been strangled when they wedge their heads in the space between the (extended) footrest and the chair: Their body weight forces the footrest down, and they choke. A safer choice, if you want this kind of chair, is the type that has no gap between the seat and the footrest.

Since you'll probably keep it a long time, don't buy a glider or rocking chair upholstered or otherwise decorated with baby themes. Get something that fits in with your other furniture.

One feature that rocker and glider fans find invaluable: Padded armrests. Once the baby grows long enough to press his feet against the chair's arms, he'll kick and catch his feet in the space between the seat and the armrest, or push against the armrest to bounce as he nurses—without unlatching.

As for nursing footrests: They're nice, but not crucial. If cost is an issue, you can press a stepstool into service. Or nail a board to two 3-inch wood blocks (4-inch blocks, if you're tall), and you'll end up with a primitive but inexpensive version of the same thing.

Routine, Difficulty with

Q: My 12-week-old son has been breastfed since day 1. He gains weight and has plenty of wet diapers, but there's no rhythm to his feeding. Sometimes he nurses every 40 minutes; last week he could go 3 hours between feeds. I've tried putting him on a schedule, but he only cries, and I end up nursing him anyway. Should he be so changeable?

A: Babies rarely cooperate with schedules or routines. The only thing that's predictable is their unpredictability! At 12 weeks, your son may be going through a growth spurt, prompting him to nurse more frequently than usual. Babies are hungrier during growth spurts, and this is especially noticeable in breastfed babies because breast milk is so swiftly digested. Formula is less easily digested, so formula-fed babies may not want to be fed as often as breastfed babies. Hang in there. If you're hopelessly tired, get into bed and take a nursing holiday. Growth spurts don't last long, and when he gets through this one, his eating schedule will be less frenetic.

See also Feeding Schedules; Schedules for Feeding and Infant Management Programs, About

Running and Breastfeeding

Q: I'd like to resume my daily runs, now that my baby's here and our breastfeeding is established. But my running partner told me that she'd heard the hormones stimulated by aerobic exercise can make breast milk taste bad. Is she right? I'd really like to get back in shape, but not at my baby's expense.

A: Your friend may be referring to a 1992 report about an Indiana University study of 26 nursing mothers who expressed milk before and after 30 minutes of vigorous exercise. Several of the babies refused the postexercise milk, and the report's authors hypothesized that the rejection was caused by higher levels of lactic acid in the breast milk. Critics of the report noted that the samples of milk were given by bottle, and since many babies accustomed to breastfeeding won't accept a bottle, the hypothesis is flawed. The babies' rejection could have been caused by the container rather than its contents.

It is true that lactic acid levels in breast milk are higher after exercise. Some babies don't mind. If yours does, you can schedule your runs to take place between nursing sessions—breastfeed first, and then run. The extra lactic acid in your breast milk will dissipate within an hour after you finish exercising.

Before resuming your running program, make sure your physician agrees. You'll also want an extra-supportive exercise bra. Drink plenty of water to replace what you lose when you sweat.

See also Exercise and Breastfeeding

Rusty Pipe Syndrome

Q: I am 32 weeks pregnant and have noticed a pinkish discharge from my nipples. It first looked like pink-tinged colostrum, but after I expressed some, the discharge turned dark red, like blood. Could you explain this?

A: It may be a condition informally known as rusty pipe syndrome, which is generally harmless to an expectant mom, or to a baby if the discharge appears after the baby is born. The discharge probably is colostrum, in your case. Rusty pipe syndrome also shows up in lactating mothers.

Blood in your colostrum or breast milk can be traced to several causes. If it occurs in late pregnancy or in the early postpartum period, it may be caused by a harmless breast tumor called an intraductal papilloma. If that's what it is, you're likely to notice pinkish colostrum or breast milk in only one breast. An intraductal papilloma is too small to be felt as a lump. Usually, it's accompanied by discomfort or pain in that breast.

Another possible cause: broken capillary veins within the

breast. Capillaries are delicate and can be broken if your breast is massaged too vigorously, or if you're using a breast pump improperly (setting it too high or too fast, for example, or failing to center your breast).

Talk to your OB/GYN or health care provider about the discharge, just to be on the safe side. You'll feel better, and if there is a problem, it's better to address it now than later.

See also Pumping, About

Scales

Q: When the pediatrician weighed my 7-month-old son at his office, he registered almost a pound lighter than on our home scale. Could his scale be wrong?

A: Yes. So could yours. Scales vary, sometimes dramatically, from one to another. But what's more relevant is what your son weighs in comparison to his last weight at the pediatrician's office (assuming that the pediatrician is using the same scale). If your health maintenance organization bounces you around to different pediatricians and different offices, express your worries, and ask if your son can be weighed on another scale to get a better idea of his true weight. How about other measurements—his head circumference, height, and developmental milestones? Older breastfed babies (6 to 12 months old) tend to be long and lean compared with formula-fed babies. A younger baby who's lean is probably not getting enough milk. But if your son really is underweight and is lagging behind in other categories, talk to your pediatrician about examining the possible causes of those delays.

See also Weight and Growth Charts, About

Schedules for Feeding and Infant Management Programs, About
Rigid feeding schedules were first developed at the beginning of the 20th century, when psychologists and physicians decided that babies should be reared according to strict rules. Hospitals adopted schedules primarily for their staff's convenience when formula—which takes nearly twice as long as breast milk for a baby to digest—became available at about the same time.

By the 1990s, hospitals began reevaluating feeding schedules, especially for babies whose mothers planned to breastfeed. Several studies found that babies who were restricted to breastfeeding schedules during the early postpartum days had difficulty breastfeeding and that their mothers turned to formula by the time the babies were 4 to 6 weeks old.

More recently, schedules advocating feeding babies every 2-1/2 to 4 hours have become popular again, particularly in response to Gary Ezzo's Preparation for Parenting Christian education classes, and *On Becoming Babywise,* the book Ezzo coauthored with a pediatrician who took his Preparation for Parenting classes. (Ezzo is a pastor and the head of Growing Families International, a conservative Christian organization. His wife, Ann Marie, had 2 years of experience as a nurse at Concord Hospital in Concord, New Hampshire, in the 1970s.) Early editions of the *Preparation for Parenting* and *Babywise* books urge keeping babies on feeding schedules directed by the parents, not by the baby's needs. (One edition of *Babywise* instructs parents that if a baby fails to eat at one feeding, "then make her wait until the next one.") The books recommend feeding newborns no longer than 30 minutes at intervals of 2-1/2 to 3-1/2 hours, described as 2-1/2 to 3 hours from the end of the last 30-minute feeding.

Ezzo has advised parents to avoid following any schedule too rigidly—"hyperscheduling," in his phrase. However, many parents choose to interpret his program strictly, allowing their babies to cry and wait until the clock says that it's time to eat.

Recent editions of the books have been modified to more closely reflect the American Academy of Pediatrics' feeding recommendations: "Newborns should be nursed whenever they show signs of hunger, such as increased alertness or activity, mouthing or rooting. Crying is a late indicator of hunger. Newborns should be nursed approximately 8 to 12 times every 24 hours, until satiety."

The *Preparation for Parenting* and *On Becoming Babywise* advice is controversial among many pediatricians and early childhood experts. Several cases of babies suffering from failure to thrive and dehydration have resulted when parents closely follow the books' advice. So many pediatricians voiced specific concerns about the Ezzo materials that the AAP adopted a resolution to monitor the Ezzo programs.

Strict feeding schedules may work for some babies, but they often present problems, especially for breastfed babies. A mother who strictly adheres to a rigid feeding schedule risks compromising her baby's health and development, and her own milk supply. Breastfeeding successfully relies on demand and supply. Your breasts respond to the baby's needs. If you fail to feed your baby when she's hungry because it's "not time" for her to eat, your milk supply will dwindle. Growth spurts, teething, and developmental milestones all prompt babies to nurse more frequently than usual because their caloric needs skyrocket.

Scheduled Feedings

Q: I've been told to feed our new baby on my schedule, not his, and to limit the amount of time I feed—20 minutes per session one week, 10 the next—until the baby has adjusted to eating at certain times and is sleeping all night. Most of my friends who use this program have their babies on formula. Will it work with breastfed babies, too?

A: Programs that involve a structured feeding and sleeping schedule tend to be incompatible with breastfeeding. The American Academy of Pediatrics guidelines advise breastfeeding mothers to nurse babies on demand, not according to a schedule, especially during the first 2 months of life. A breastfed baby seems to digest its food much more quickly than a formula-fed baby does.

Limiting the amount of time you nurse, and the number of feedings per day, can wreak havoc on your milk supply and can dehydrate your baby if she should have a weak suck or a small tummy.

See also Ezzo, Gary; Schedules for Feeding and Infant Management Programs, About

Science of Breast Milk, About the

Even formula companies acknowledge that breast milk is better for babies than formula. Scores of studies find that breastfed babies are healthier than babies who are given formula. They're less likely than formula-fed babies to suffer from meningitis or from infections of the ear and gut, or of the respiratory or urinary tracts.

Mother's milk strengthens a newborn's defenses against foreign organisms, including disease-causing viruses and bacteria. The antibodies, proteins, and immune cells in breast milk neutralize microbes or mark them for destruction. Once ingested, the beneficial molecules and cells in breast milk help prevent microorganisms from invading the baby's body. The antibodies in breast milk are known as IgG, IgM, IgD, IgA, and IgE. The most abundant antibody is IgA, which seems to help a breastfed baby battle ingested pathogens until the baby can make IgA on her own. The IgA molecules are custom-tailored to each baby's immediate environment. A breastfeeding mother synthesizes antibodies when she comes into contact with a disease-causing agent. Each antibody she makes is specific to that agent, so the baby receives the protection she needs most. Researchers don't know how the mother's immune system knows how to distinguish between "bad" bacteria and the "good" bacteria that normally live in the gut, but the IgA molecules help ward off disease without causing an inflammation that potentially can damage an infant's delicate, developing body.

Breast milk also contains mucins, large molecules that contain a lot of protein and carbohydrate and that glom onto bacteria and viruses to eliminate them from a baby's body. The lactoferrin molecules in breast milk also help halt the spread of the disease-causing bacteria that thrive on iron. And a breastfed baby utilizes more of the iron in breast milk—about 50 percent—than a bottle-fed baby absorbs from formula. That means that a breastfed baby's gut has less available iron for bacteria than does a formula-fed baby. Bifidus factor, one of the oldest known disease-resisting elements in breast milk, helps promote the growth of a beneficial organism, *Lactobacillus bifidus,* and the free fatty acids in breast milk can fight viruses, including chicken pox. Breastfed babies produce higher levels of antibodies in response to immunization vaccines.

Scuba Diving

Q: Our family, including our 4-month-old, will vacation in Hawaii, and I'd like to go scuba diving. Could the change in pressure associated with diving affect my breast milk?

A: Not really. A negligible amount of dissolved nitrogen may be secreted in your milk, but not enough to cause concern. Do be careful to stay well hydrated. As an experienced scuba diver, you know that dehydration can cause decompression illness. Contact the Diver's Alert Network, a nonprofit organization at Duke University Medical Center, if you have other questions about diving (910–684–2948).

Sex and Breastfeeding, About

Moms who've spent most of the past 24 hours caring for a baby tend to view sex quite differently from fathers who work outside the home. (It's like the split-scene in *Annie Hall* when the therapists each ask how often the couple has sex: "All the time! At least three times a week," the woman tells her therapist. "Almost never! Maybe three times a week," the man complains to his.)

Sometimes breastfeeding decreases a woman's libido. Sometimes breastfeeding speeds it up. Sexual desire is complicated and unpredictable for new parents. Their intimate time is eclipsed. They're often exhausted, especially the mother, who finds her life orbiting around her baby's.

A new mom tends to be "touched out": she spends so much time holding, nursing, burping, and carrying the baby, and attending to any older children, that she may see sex as yet another demand on her time and body. When you're touched out, solitude is infinitely more appealing than sex. (For a woman who feels touched out, a long bath alone, while Dad takes the baby and any siblings out of the house for an hour or so, is the equivalent of foreplay. Works better than a dozen roses.)

When a couple finally does get some intimate time together, both partners need to understand that a lactating woman often lacks vaginal lubrication, even when she's sexually aroused. Hormones, not libido, are to blame. (Try commercial lubricants.)

Here's what one new father had to say about sex life A.B. (After Baby):

"We had a little girl about 4 months ago, and we are just barely getting back to what is, in my opinion, a normal-to-decent sex life. As the male here, I guess my wife feels I've been somewhat pushy. It's a little bit of a shock to have to slow or slow so much, but things get better, if you're patient.

"It's frustrating for me, and for my wife, too. She wants to satisfy me, and herself, but if she's sore or 'touched out,' we're just out of luck. The best thing to do, when you can't have old-fashioned sex, is to try other forms of it—cuddling, the kind of heavy foreplay that got us hot in high school, masturbation (if that works for you), and oral sex.

"My wife still feels a little out of synch—that her body's not attractive, and it's hard for her to get in the mood. She worries. From my point of view, I can't get enough of her. So what if she's got a little pouchy after pregnancy? It's a nice, soft spot to nestle against. Keep a good frame of mind. Humor and patience help."

Need a head start on humor? Here's one mom's list of how breastfeeding is like sex:

- Bodily fluids all over your clothes and/or sheets afterward.
- Unthinkable with someone you're not extremely close to.
- Less pleasant in extremely hot or cold weather.
- Once you're used to it, you get irritable when you miss it for a while.
- Requires engorgement on the part of at least one party.
- One of you tends to roll over and fall asleep afterward.
- Can be done in various positions.
- Can be done in bed or out.
- Lots of people need training and practice to get the hang of it.
- People ask you nosy questions about it.
- If you can't do it, there are substitutes, but many people find them less satisfying.

Sex, Avoiding?

Q: My mother told me that nursing women should not have sexual intercourse. She says it will sour the milk. I thought she was ridiculous (and intrusive!), but the morning after my husband and I celebrated the end of 6-week postpartum celibacy, my baby was exceptionally gassy and fussy. Does sex affect breast milk?

A: Stimulation and orgasm can trigger your letdown reflex. Otherwise, sex doesn't affect the flavor or composition of breast milk. If you've got the energy and inclination, go ahead!

By the way, if you're curious about the source of your mom's theory, it could be herbalist Jethro Kloss, author of *Back to Eden: The Classic Guide to Herbal Medicine, Natural Foods and Home Remedies* (Woodbridge Press; originally published in 1939, reprinted in 1972). Kloss combined sensible advice—pureed fruits and vegetables for first solids, gradual weaning, lots of water to maintain a good milk supply—with eyebrow-raising claims. A relevant sample: "Two of the most important things when nursing a child is to keep the bowels regular and the mother should be calm at all times. Sexual intercourse, during this time, often causes children to have colic and stomach trouble, as it has a damaging effect on the milk because of the excitement."

Sex and Night Feedings

Q: Our 17-month-old daughter goes to bed after nursing at 7:30 P.M. and then is up again at 10 P.M. and again at 4 A.M. Her 10 P.M. wake-up and feeding is the problem. My husband and I have little time alone together anyway, and this is throwing a big wrench in our sex life. I know eventually she'll sleep, but meantime, how can my husband and I get some "grown-up" time together without one eye on the clock?

A: You've got a lot of company. Most couples find their sex life is pretty slim pickin's during the first 2 years after a baby is born. There's an inverse correlation between a baby's energy and his parents'. Between their exhaustion and the baby's erratic sleep patterns (growth spurts, teething, ear infections, etc.), many parents find that one is too pooped to party, or that when they're both amorous, that's when the baby decides to wake up.

One solution, given your baby's age, is to try feeding her two mini-dinners instead of one dinner before the 7:30 P.M. nursing session. Some parents find that babies sleep longer when they eat a light dinner in the early evening (between 5 and 6 P.M.), and a second dinner about an hour or two later. Try feeding her baby foods, like meat, that take a long time to digest. That may help her sleep beyond 10 P.M.

And don't discount the value of a quickie. It can help open your hearts and jump-start a flagging romance. Brevity can be as titillating, and sexually rewarding, for women as it is for men.

See also Sex and Breastfeeding, About

Sexuality: Is Breastfeeding Erotic?

Q: My wife breastfeeds our baby daughter. I've read that breastfeeding stimulates the sort of endorphins that make you happy. She says nursing is physically satisfying, but I also wonder whether nursing is sexually stimulating. "Wouldn't it be like foreplay?" I asked my wife, but she only rolled her eyes.

A: Oh, yeah, especially if you're turned on by cracked nipples and painfully engorged breasts, and your secret fantasy is being a 24-hour milk bar. (Seriously: some women do experience sexual feelings while nursing. It's normal, but uncommon.)

Most women find an enormous difference between breastfeeding a baby and being nuzzled by a sex partner. When a baby latches on correctly, the nursing mom feels only a distant tugging sensation that is more clinical than erotic. When a baby latches on incorrectly, the mom typically feels an excruciating pain that is definitely not erotic. For most women, nursing a baby is not in the same league as foreplay.

Showers and Letdown

Q: When I take a shower—which sometimes isn't until 9 P.M. these days!—my milk starts letting down. If the baby's awake and crying, the flow won't stop, and I worry about wasting her milk. What can I do to stop it?

A: You're not losing enough milk in the shower to affect your baby's nutrition, so don't worry about that. A lot of nursing moms find that their milk lets down in the shower—it's stimulated by the warm water. (Baths and hot tubs have the same effect.) If it bothers you, press a damp washcloth firmly against your nipples, and the flow will stop, or at least slow down.

If you're tired of waiting for hours to shower, bring your baby into the bathroom with you. You can put an infant in a car seat or a bouncy seat on the floor or, after her neck muscles are stronger, hang a johnny jump-up from the door frame so the baby can see you. An older baby can sit outside the shower, or you can bring your baby in the tub with you, at the far end, in a tub seat with a few bath toys. Rinse carefully to avoid accidentally splashing soapy water into the baby's face.

Siblings, Nursing

Q: I have a 3-year-old who self-weaned at 20 months, and I'm expecting a baby next month. We've looked at books of babies and babies nursing to prepare him for the baby's birth. Now my son is expressing an interest in nursing again—not now, but after the baby is born. How do I handle this?

A: Many siblings react to a new baby sister or brother by reverting to baby behavior themselves. By preparing your son for the new baby, and what to expect at the baby's feeding time, you've already got a head start.

Your 3-year-old may want to nurse—it's fairly common for older siblings to ask for your milk. (Older siblings may also go back to baby talk and want to be held like an infant, and even ask to wear diapers or sleep in the crib.)

How about suggesting that once the baby is born, and your milk supply is established, your son can taste your milk that's been expressed into a cup? (Don't take it personally if he doesn't like it. Few older children find warm breast milk appealing.)

If he still wants to nurse, and if you decide to allow him to nurse, remember that it's been a while since he's suckled. He may not remember how, though he'll probably be able to elicit enough to get a taste. If he decides breast milk is yucky, case closed. But he may decide that he likes it, and you'll find yourself tandem-nursing a toddler and a newborn.

If that's not appealing, try distracting him. Plan some activities for him when it's the baby's feeding time—maybe playing with water, or clay, or allowing him to write with a pen (a big deal for toddlers) or watch a favorite video. Plan a lot of nonnursing cuddling time, so he knows that you love him as much as you love the baby.

See also Tandem Nursing

Silicone Implants

Q: I have silicone implants in my breasts, placed there about 10 years ago. My surgeon told me I wouldn't be able to breastfeed, but my obstetrician says that I may be able to nurse. I'm worried that the milk might be tainted by the silicone, or that I may not produce enough milk.

A: Many women who've had breast implants are able to nurse their babies. Silicone implants are compatible with breastfeeding.

There is a 1.5 percent chance that your implants could leak. However, silicone is not absorbed into the gastrointestinal tract. If the silicone does leak, its high molecular weight makes it unlikely that it could get into your alveoli—the milk-producing cells.

Work with a certified lactation consultant who can show you the best nursing positions and help evaluate your milk supply.

The only way to know whether you can produce enough milk is to breastfeed your baby. If she is producing the appropriate number of wet and poopy diapers (*see* Diaper Count), then she is getting enough. As your milk comes in she should have six to eight wet diapers and one or two stools a day. If her diaper count is normal and her weight gain is on target, you'll be fine. Even if she's not producing enough diapers and you need to supplement, you can continue nursing. Breastfeeding is as much an act of nurturing as feeding.

See also Dehydration; Lactation Consultant

Simethicone Drops

Q: What is simethicone? A friend told me that I should give my baby simethicone drops to counter the effects of my overactive letdown.

A: Simethicone is the generic name for anti-gas treatments. If you have an overactive letdown, the baby may be gulping a lot of air and swallowing more foremilk than hindmilk, which results in gas and irritability. However, giving her simethicone treats the symptom, not the cause. To address both, make the appropriate changes in your nursing routine, and give your baby the antigas drops until the situation improves.

See also Overactive Letdown

Sippy Cups vs. Bottles

Q: My baby is 6 months old and exclusively breastfed, and she is, to put it mildly, not receptive to taking a bottle. She won't suck on a bottle at all. She gets in a screaming frenzy when my mother or my husband tries to give her a bottle when I'm gone. I'm going back to work, and I'm worrying that she'll never take a bottle. What can I do?

A: Since your daughter is an older baby, you might be better off going to a sippy cup. Settled babies who've never had a bottle often seem to find it easier to use a sippy cup. Try her on a spill-proof cup, and on a non-spillproof cup. Sometimes babies find the non-spillproof version easier to use. Many breastfed babies make the transition to sippy cups more readily than they do to bottles. Avent's soft-spout sippy cup is especially popular with nursing moms.

One downside of sippy cups: Some babies are more interested in teething on the spouts than in drinking from them. Give these babies water, not expressed milk, in sippy cups. Otherwise, you'll cringe when you see that hard-won breast milk dribbling from his chin as he gnaws on the spout.

Another downside: Even the "spillproof" sippy cups do spill, with or without the lid on.

See also Bottle, Refusing

Sleeping and Nursing

Q: I'm in tears, and it's 3:30 A.M. My 6-month-old wakes up at 11 P.M., 2 A.M., and 4 or 4:30 A.M. to nurse. I've tried cutting out night feedings cold turkey, but I can't tolerate her crying. So I get up and nurse her, but I can't keep this up forever. Help!

A: Sleep is precious to new moms. Have you found a nursing position that allows you to doze or sleep while you're securely holding the baby? A family bed—the baby sleeping with you and your husband—can minimize your sleep deprivation. Some moms can nurse when they're lying down, but others, especially well-endowed mothers, find that difficult. If you do use a family bed, make sure you block any gaps where the baby could be trapped.

An alternative to family beds: a comfortable recliner, which provides support and security. The football hold is best if you're nursing in a recliner.

Whichever you choose, make sure your back is supported. It should be at a 45-degree angle (/ or \), not 90 degrees. Remember to lift your breast up to your baby's head.

See also Positions, About

Sleep Habits, Changes in

Q: My 4-month-old son began sleeping through the night (6 to 9 hours at a stretch) when he was 9 weeks old. But last week, he started waking up, ravenous, 4 hours after I put him down. I fed him, but he woke up 2 hours later. I'm exhausted. What should I do? Put him on a routine?

A: Three things wreak havoc with a baby's sleep at night: teething, ear infections, and growth spurts. If it were an ear infection, you'd probably know right away—he'd be screaming inconsolably, and might have a fever as well. If you suspect an ear infection, take him to a doctor. Some babies tolerate pain more stoically than others, and ear infections can result in permanent hearing damage.

Could he be teething? Is he drooling a lot? Chewing on his fist or toys? Most babies get their first tooth between 4 and 6 months of age. Teething is very painful—enough to wake babies up at night.

If he's going through a growth spurt, putting him on a schedule probably won't change his behavior. He may go back to his former sleep habits in a week or so when the growth spurt concludes, the tooth cuts through, or the antibiotics for an ear infection take effect.

Some babies respond well to routines and schedules, but

going by the clock can be disastrous for other babies. Growth spurts and illnesses toss most schedules out the window.
See also Ear Infection; Scheduled Feedings; Growth Spurts, About; Teething and Nursing

Sleep, Disassociating from Breastfeeding

Q: My 10-month-old son sometimes will go to sleep if we put him down when he's drowsy, but usually he has to be nursed until he calms down enough to sleep. He's capable of staying alert longer than I am. How can I get him to go to sleep without nursing?

A: Have you tried shifting the last nursing session to about 30 minutes before bedtime, so he's not hungry but is satiated? Has your spouse tried taking over the bedtime routine? Babies have extremely sensitive noses—your son may want to nurse just because he can smell your milk.

You may want to establish a new bedtime ritual focused on other things—bedtime stories, lullabies, reading favorite bedtime stories like *Goodnight Moon, Good Night, Gorilla,* or *Dr. Seuss' ABC* until you find one that holds his interest. If he keeps nursing, try a variation on the *Goodnight Moon* theme: Hold him, and walk around the house, or his room, saying goodnight to everything—including appliances.

Look for other good suggestions in parenting books. Dr. William Sears' *The Fussy Baby: How to Bring Out the Best in Your High-Needs Child* and his *Nighttime Parenting* are especially helpful. And if nothing else works, remember this: Nursing a baby to sleep isn't wrong. It's normal. He won't be a baby forever.

Sleepy Baby, and Difficulty Nursing

Q: Help! My 5-day-old daughter always falls asleep while nursing. She'll suck for 5 minutes, then fall asleep, wake up, suck, and then sleep again. Last night it took an hour and a half to get through nursing her—and then we had to wake her up again 30 minutes later. How can we get her to stay awake?

A: You're not alone. Newborns, like new moms, tend to be sleepy for the first few days or even the first couple of weeks. Some parents find that nursing is a two-person job: Mom lies on the bed while Dad holds the baby to the nipple.

Try these strategies to keep her awake:

- Strip her down to a diaper, so she's a bit cool; sleepy babies may be more alert with skin-to-skin contact. Drape a receiving blanket around both of you if you're chilly.
- Try breast compression to keep your milk flowing; babies tend to fall asleep when the flow slows, and a fast flow of milk keeps them awake and fills them up.
- Wake her gently by laying her along your forearms, facing you, and bring her slowly upright; repeat until she looks at you.
- Softly repeat her name.
- Every five or six sucks, or whenever she starts to slow down, stimulate her by touching her chin or gently moving her head.
- Stroke and tickle her arms, legs, feet, or ears when she starts to nod off.
- Switch sides when she loses interest in feeding.
- Sing a lively song—not a lullaby, but something you danced to in high school.
- Wipe her gently with a cool, damp washcloth, or give her a bath.

And schedule a visit with your pediatrician. She'll want to make sure the baby's weight gain is on target, and look at your daughter herself.

See also Breast Compression; Burping a Sleepy Baby; Switch Nursing

Slings and Breastfeeding

Q: My 8-week-old loves to be carried but seems to hate being in a sling, a Snugli, or any other kind of baby wrap. I've tried the sling on and off since she was born, but to no avail. I thought it would be perfect for discreet breastfeeding, but she hates it. What are we doing wrong?

A: If you're using the sling properly—ask another sling-wearer for help—the answer probably lies in your baby's age rather than in your sling-carrying technique. Very young infants often dislike slings and their cousins—Baby Wraps, Snuglis, etc. Try again after your baby is a little older (10 weeks to 3 months). If the sling seems too big, it's the wrong type or size. It's also possible that your 8-week-old may be ready to sit in a front carrier and look at her new world.

See also Baby Carriers, About; Breastfeeding in Public, About

Small Breasts

Q: I am very small-breasted. Totally flat, actually. Some of my better-endowed friends tell me I won't be able to nurse when I have a baby. I'm already 24 and still have an AA cup. Will I be able to breastfeed?

A: Many small-breasted women, especially if they have an inferiority complex about their breast size, worry about the same thing—often needlessly. Breast size is unrelated to your ability to produce milk. One mom who wore an AAA cup tandem-nursed her twins, with no supply problems. "The unexpected benefit of that," she said, "was that I have a newfound pride in my breasts, and it has nothing to do with their appearance! They are amazing and super-efficient, and my two wonderful babies are proof of that."

Smoke, Secondhand

Q: My husband and I are bringing our 2-month-old son to spend the holidays with my in-laws. I'm worried because they're all chain-smokers, and we'll be staying in their home for more than a week. What effect will exposure to secondhand smoke have on my son and on my milk supply?

A: Smokers inhale only 15 percent of a cigarette's smoke. The other 85 percent goes into the air as secondhand smoke. Secondhand smoke contains more than 4,000 chemicals, including at least 40 carcinogens. If you are constantly exposed to secondhand smoke, you'll passively inhale the equivalent of two or three cigarettes a day. Secondhand smoke is linked to more than 10,000 hospitalizations of infants and children each year. (For more information, *see* Resources to contact the Centers for Disease Control for its publication *Secondhand Smoke in your Home.*)

A week of constant exposure to secondhand smoke probably will compromise your family's health, especially if you have a history of asthma or other respiratory illnesses. Secondhand smoke is a contributing factor in ear infections and lung disorders. It also can affect your breast milk. A 1983 study found that nicotine easily enters the breast milk of even nonsmokers who are steadily exposed to cigarette smoke. It may diminish your supply.

Ask if your hosts are willing to establish nonsmoking rooms, especially the rooms where you'll spend a lot of time. If they're reluctant, you may want to choose alternative accommodations.

Smoking and Breastfeeding

Q: I know I should stop smoking, but I can't. Will the chemicals from the smoke I inhale get into my breast milk? Is it better to give my 5-week-old son formula?

A: No. As you know, your baby's health, and your own, will be better if you can shake the cigarette habit. Heavy smokers produce less milk than nonsmokers, and their milk has exceptionally low levels of vitamin C. Smoking increases your baby's risk for gastroesophageal reflux, sudden infant death syndrome, allergies, bronchitis, colic, diarrhea, and other disorders. In a 1937 study, nicotine addiction was diagnosed in an infant whose mother smoked heavily. The American Medical Association's position paper on secondhand smoke places it as a Class A carcinogen, the same category as asbestos and benzene.

If you can't quit smoking, breastfeeding is still superior to formula. Try to breastfeed as long as possible. Studies have shown that smokers' breastfed babies are healthier than smokers' formula-fed babies. Your breast milk will help counter the smoke's negative effects. In short, it's better to smoke and breastfeed than to smoke and formula-feed.

If you want to quit smoking, it is safe to use nicotine patches while you're breastfeeding. The dose of nicotine is lower than you consume while smoking—and if a patch can help you quit, so much the better for you and for your baby.

Soap, Using on Breasts

Q: My sister told me that I shouldn't use soap, lotion, or powder because I breastfeed. Why not? And how do I keep clean? In the shower, I can't avoid getting soap and shampoo on my breasts.

A: Don't worry about that. The shampoo and soap will rinse off. On the other hand, if you rub soap into your breasts and nipples, it may dry them out and facilitate cracked nipples—something you'd rather read about than experience; trust me. Lactating breasts make their own cleaning, moisturizing substance. All you really need to do is rinse them with clean water. (How dirty could they be, anyway?)

It is a good idea to avoid putting lotions and powders on your breasts. Some is bound to get on your nipples, and your baby probably won't like the flavor. Even if she doesn't mind that, the chemicals in those products won't do her any favors.

Soft Breasts

Q: I've been nursing my baby for 7 weeks. Just a few days ago, she stopped her almost nonstop nursing at night and started sleeping 6 hours or so. I was engorged when I woke up, and she nursed fine. But later she slept through a couple of feedings, and instead of getting engorged, my breasts seemed very soft, as if they were empty. Am I losing my milk?

A: Probably not. If your baby has nursed so steadily since birth, missing a feed or two shouldn't interfere with your supply. Is she producing the right number of soaked and poopy diapers? (*See* Diaper Count.) Do you hear sucking and swallowing sounds when she does nurse? Do you see her jaw and/or temple wiggling? Do you allow her to end nursing sessions instead of pulling her off the breast? Those are indications of a sufficient supply.

Let your baby suckle for comfort as well as for nutrition. Follow her cues. When she roots around, or tries to suck on her fist or something else, pop open your nursing bra. Have a nursing holiday, when you and the baby spend the day in bed (or on the sofa), doing nothing but nursing and snoozing.

See also Supply Problems, About

Soft Drinks

Q: I eat right, and I drink a lot of water (8 ounces, four or five times a day), but I also like to drink colas. I've been drinking the caffeine-free diet kind. Sometimes I drink more diet cola than water, even though I suspect I shouldn't. Is there a reason I should limit the number of soft drinks I consume?

A: Well, they're not doing you much good, nutritionally speaking. A bigger concern with diet soft drinks is aspartame, the artificial sweetener typically used in commercial diet drinks. NutraSweet and other artificial sweeteners are controversial. The jury's still out on whether they're potentially harmful, but why risk it? Try cutting down to one or two diet sodas a day.

Have you tried herbal iced teas? Even nursing moms who usually don't like tea find that herbal iced teas make an acceptable substitute for soft drinks. Sample the spiced teas and fruit teas, or combine flavors, until you find something you like. Bottled water is another good substitute; it has the convenience of bottled soft drinks but is superior nutritionally.

See also Caffeine, Effects on Breast Milk

Solids, Breastfed Baby Refusing

Q: We've tried introducing solids, on and off, since my son was almost 4 months old. We started by mixing rice cereal with expressed breast milk. He never took more than a teaspoon, and then only when it was mostly breast milk with a few dissolved rice flakes.

Now he's 5 months old. He seems interested in watching us eat, but he still won't taste more than a teaspoon or two of applesauce, pureed sweet potatoes, or other foods before he gets upset and clamps his lips together. His weight's on target, but shouldn't he be eating solids by now?

A: Many babies begin eating solids only when they're between 7 and 12 months old. As long as your son is gaining weight appropriately, and you're giving him a chance to try solids once a day, he'll be okay.

Never force a baby to eat. He'll eat when he's ready—and waiting until he shows signs of being ready for solid foods will help him avoid food allergies. The developmental window between 6 and 8 months of age is important for self-feeding, but it's normal for a baby to be wary of trying new things. The trick is to keep exploring and offering different options. Don't give up. If he starts to lose weight or shows an allergic reaction to the foods you introduce, see your pediatrician.

Solids, Increasing Appetite

Q: My 6-month-old son was exclusively breastfed until a few days ago, when he turned into an eatin' and drinkin' machine. He's hungry all the time, reaching for food on our plates even after he's had his dinner, and on top of this, he won't sleep at night. I thought once he started eating solids, he'd sleep more at night. What am I doing wrong?

A: Adding solids to your baby's diet doesn't always mean that he'll sleep through the night, especially if you're introducing solids to a very young (5 months or younger) baby. But it sounds as if you're not doing anything wrong. Babies have growth spurts at 3 weeks, at 6 weeks, and around 3 months and 6 months. If he's going through a growth spurt, his ravenous appetite will calm down in a few days.

Could he be teething? That would explain his wakefulness, along with his need to chew. If he's going through a growth spurt *and* teething, you'll need patience, fortitude, and plenty of frozen washcloths for him to gnaw on. His teeth may not push through for a few days to a week or so, and the process is painful.

See also Growth Spurts, About; Teething and Nursing

Sore Nipples

See Nipples, Sore, About

Sour/Spoiled Breast Milk

Q: I've been struggling to get our 5-month-old son to take a bottle of expressed milk while my wife's at work, without much luck. Today, he made such a face that I tasted the milk myself. Yuck. I defrosted three other bags of expressed milk—all sour. She only pumped the milk 2 days ago. What are we doing wrong?

A: Are you storing the milk in the freezer door, or in the front of the freezer? Opening and shutting the door can warm the milk enough to let it thaw enough to spoil. If you have a self-defrosting freezer, and the milk is in the back of the freezer, the defrosting mechanism could be at fault. Store bags of expressed milk in the center of the freezer, where they'll stay fresh.

The other possibility, and it's a long shot, is that your wife has excess lipase in her milk. Breast milk should taste sweet. Milk with too much lipase starts to taste repulsive almost as soon as it starts getting cooler than body temperature. If freshly expressed milk tastes worse than sour after less than 2 hours—as if it's been regurgitated—your wife may have excess lipase.

See also Lipase, Excessive; Microwave Heating Expressed Milk; Pumping, About

Spitting Up: How Much Is Too Much?

Q: My 1-month-old son often spits up after nursing. It's not a lot—maybe 1 or 2 tablespoons' worth of what looks like curdled milk—but I have no idea how much he's keeping down. How can I tell if he's eating enough? How much spit-up is too much?

A: Most young babies spit up small amounts of milk. If you're really worried, use a rubber spatula to scrape up and measure the spit-up. Usually, it's less than a tablespoon or two. (It just looks like more!) As long as he's producing enough wet and poopy diapers, he's getting enough to eat. (*See* Diaper Count.)

If he consistently spits up immediately after he nurses, and seems constantly fussy and unhappy, it could be a sign that he's allergic to something in your diet. (*See* Allergies [Baby's], About.)

If your baby is spitting up, and then gasping and struggling to breathe, have your pediatrician see him immediately to evaluate your son for the possibility of reflux. (Also often associated with reflux is stridor, a narrow airway that causes the baby to breathe noisily and in a sing-song rhythm.)

Some babies with reflux don't always spit up excessively. Instead, they re-swallow partly digested milk, and the gastric acids burn their esophagus, leaving them extremely uncomfortable, with colic-type symptoms. If it is reflux, you'll be glad you caught it early. Reflux tends to get worse as time goes on. (Well, it gets worse, and then better, and then worse again, in a nastily relentless cycle.)

See also Allergies (Baby's), Vomiting Baby and Breastfeeding; Reflux

Spoiling?

Q: My mother-in-law says I'm spoiling my 8-week-old son by holding him and nursing him so often. She tells me to let him cry at night instead of going to him. Is it possible to spoil a baby who's this young?

A: Babies need to be held and comforted, especially during the first few weeks after birth. Comforting (or trying to comfort) a crying baby is one of the most difficult and exasperating jobs of

being a new parent, but it helps teach your baby to be secure and trusting. There is no scientific evidence that an infant can be spoiled by being held or nursed frequently, and plenty of studies that show that babies benefit enormously by having their needs met. Babies who are held frequently, and whose cries are answered, cry less than babies who are ignored.
See also Schedules for Feeding and Infant Management Programs

Spraying Milk

Q: When my baby starts to nurse, she gulps and chokes at first because she gets such mouthfuls of milk. My nipples literally spray milk. If she pulls off the breast, there's a 1- to 3-foot jet of milk. The firehose effect slows down at the end. Is this normal?
A: Spraying milk is a sign of an overactive letdown, and it's common in women blessed with an ample milk supply. The milk that sprays usually is foremilk—the thinner milk. Hindmilk is heavier and more likely to ebb than spray.
See also Colic; Overactive Letdown

Stains

Q: Is there a way to get rid of old spit-up stains? I just received bags and bags of hand-me-downs that are in perfect shape, except for yellow stains around the neck area.
A: Some stains will never come out, especially if they've been heat-set by a drier. Here's a recipe that will take out almost every stain except for ballpoint ink and indelible marker:

Mix about 1 cup Cascade dishwasher detergent, 1 cup Clorox 2, and 1 gallon of water. Soak until the stain is gone; it may take a couple of hours, or it may take a week. (Alternative: Soak the garment, and leave it outside in the sun all day.) Launder as usual.

Stools, Dark, Newborn's

Q: My 5-day-old son is still having very dark stools—very green or dark brown and tarry. Is he still supposed to be passing meconium?

A: No. By the time a baby is 5 days old, his stools should be mustard-colored and seedy, not tarry. This is a sign that your baby may not be getting enough milk. Make an appointment immediately with your pediatrician, and have your son measured and weighed.

Stools, Gassy

See Allergies (Baby's), About; Colic; Foremilk and Hindmilk; Stools, Green

Stools, Green

Q: My 3-month-old son's stools have been green for almost 2 weeks. They're not foul-smelling, and tested negative for viruses and bacteria. The stool looks like normal-looking breastfed baby poop, except for the color. Is this normal?

A: Mustard-yellow to greenish stools are within the normal range. If the stools are very green, there may be a hindmilk/foremilk imbalance. If that's the cause, you can solve it by feeding from only one breast at a time, for 4 hours or so, to make sure the baby gets the calorie-rich hindmilk and not too much foremilk, which can have a laxative effect.

Often, a hindmilk/foremilk imbalance occurs when a mom has a very abundant milk supply, or if the baby is switched from one breast to the other according to a schedule, or if the baby fails to get a good latch-on. The green stools and gas are caused by too much lactose—and high-volume, low-calorie foremilk is full of lactose. A baby who is getting too much foremilk usually wants to eat frequently or for long periods of time (more than 20 minutes per breast). He's always hungry because he fills up (and empties out) quickly, and he's gassy because when the extra lactose reaches his colon, it ferments and causes gas, colic, and frothy, acid-green stools.

The solution: Let the baby control his nursing session. Forget about the clock. When you're nursing, let your son end the first breast on his own, when he's relaxed and satisfied. If he's properly positioned and latched on, and getting a good mouthful of your breast, let him nurse as long as he wants. (It's fine to let him nurse on one side per feeding, if that's all he wants.) If the other breast feels uncomfortably engorged, express a little until it feels more like a breast than a watermelon.

See also Allergies (Baby's), About; Colic; Positions, About; Spraying Milk

Stools, Infrequent

Q: My 3-month-old son is exclusively breastfed. Last week, he went 4 days without a bowel movement, and then he pooped up to his ears—literally! Should we be giving him suppositories?

A: It's not unusual for a baby (6 weeks old or more) who's exclusively breastfed to go for long periods of time—2 to 10 days—without producing a stool. As long as your son seems comfortable, happy, and alert between bowel movements, and he's producing lots of wet (not yellow) diapers, don't worry. Suppositories are unnecessary.

The general rule is that a 1-day-old newborn will produce one stool; a 2-day-old baby will produce two stools; a 3-day-old baby will produce three stools; and a 4-day-old baby will produce four stools. After that, your milk should be in, and a baby will poop at least four times a day. A baby under 3 months old should produce a lot of stools. If he doesn't, it means he is not getting enough to eat. It is not unusual for an older baby (3 months plus) to go 2 or 3 days before producing a stool. (And that one makes up for all the days he missed.) However, if his stools are little more than a stain on his diaper, he may not be getting enough milk. Take him immediately to your pediatrician to have him weighed.

Stools, Painful and Gassy

Q: My 11-week-old girl seems to be in pain when she has bowel movements. She has explosive, gassy BMs! My husband calls them volcanic poops. Sometimes it's a blowout that requires a bath. Is this due to something I'm eating?

A: It may just be her immature digestive system getting under way. If her stools are gassy only sometimes, try to analyze what you've eaten in the past 6 hours. Does she have other symptoms of a dairy sensitivity? (*See* Allergies [Baby's], About.)

It's also possible that she's getting too much foremilk and not enough hindmilk. The high-lactose foremilk makes babies gassy.

See also Allergies, Dairy; Foremilk and Hindmilk

Stools While Nursing

Q: My son almost always passes a stool when he's breastfeeding. Is this normal?

A: Yes, even though it can be disconcerting. Suckling can prompt the bowels to empty. Look at it this way: At least you can be sure that your son's wearing a clean diaper.

Stools with Blood and Mucus

Q: My 6-week-old daughter seems healthy, and she's thriving—gaining weight, and producing plenty of wet and poopy diapers. She's been exclusively breastfed. Lately I've noticed that her stools have thready, stringy mucus. Sometimes the thread of mucus looks pink or red. The pediatrician can find nothing wrong with her—no parasites or anything. Could something be wrong with my milk?

A: The stools you're describing could indicate an overactive letdown and/or a foremilk/hindmilk imbalance. (*See* Foremilk and Hindmilk.) If it's accompanied by other symptoms, the problem may be a food sensitivity. Make sure your pediatrician sees a stool sample to verify whether blood is present. If it is, the problem may be in your diet. The most common culprit is dairy products. (*See* Allergies [Baby's], About.)

Storing and Freezing Expressed Milk

See Pumping, About: Storing and Using Expressed Milk

Strike, Nursing

See Nursing Strike

Suck, Poor or Ineffective

Q: My 7-week-old son spent his first 2 weeks in the pediatric intensive care unit, being treated for hypoglycemia and other problems. I stayed there to nurse him and continued to breastfeed after he came home. But he's not gaining enough weight, even though I feed on demand. The lactation consultant says he has a poor suck reflex. What can I do to overcome this?

A: Your son may benefit from seeing a speech pathologist, who can suggest some exercises and techniques to improve your son's suck reflex. You may want to supplement his feedings with expressed milk using a tube feeding lactation aid, although that system has its drawbacks for babies with suck difficulties: If a baby can't suck well, pouring more milk into his mouth can be dangerous.

Have a lactation consultant analyze your letdown. It's possible that your son is nursing well at the beginning, when your letdown is strong, but resorts to passive suckling once the initial flow slows. You may want to try encouraging your letdown with breast compression as you nurse.

See also Breast Compression; Finger Feeding; Lactation Consultant; Tube Feeding Lactation Aid

Sucking Constantly

Q: My 3-week-old wants to suckle all the time, even after he's drained every drop of breast milk. I know that suckling is normal, natural, and healthy, but I wish he'd discover his fingers! My mom says I should let him nurse only when he's actually eating. Is it OK to let them suckle when they just want to suck?

A: Most babies go through a growth spurt when they're about 3 weeks old. Often, they're ravenous and wakeful and need to suck for both nutrition and comfort. In a few days, he'll settle down again. In the meantime, he may want to be held a lot. You can see if he likes a front baby carrier, like a Snugli, or a baby sling. If he likes a baby carrier, you can nurse him, even in public, and nobody (except for you and the baby) will be the wiser.

Comfort-nursing is as important as nutritive nursing. There's more to breastfeeding than just milk.

See also Growth Spurts, About

Supplemental Nursing System

See Tube Feeding Lactation Aid

Supply Problems, About

Almost every mother wonders whether her milk supply is sufficient. Milk production varies not only from mother to mother but from from day to day, and even morning to evening. With a few exceptions—see "When Supply Is a Problem," below—most mothers are physically capable of making enough milk to feed her baby.

During the first days after birth, your breasts are making enough colostrum and/or milk to satisfy your baby. Colostrum only looks thin and watery—it's packed with antibodies that compose a perfect first meal. If your baby acts hungry, she may not be latched on correctly. A baby who's not fully latched on can't get at the colostrum. Odds are that if you think you have supply problems, you probably should be looking at your baby's latch and/or the baby's sucking technique.

Different conditions—a baby's growth spurt, breasts that feel soft instead of full, a baby uninterested in or apparently distressed by nursing—can give you the impression that your supply is low. Almost always, your milk production adjusts to the baby's demand.

If she's nursing more, she may be going through a growth spurt, teething, or approaching a developmental milestone.

Once you've established nursing, your breasts may not get engorged or even feel full, but as long as the baby is latched on correctly, suckling, and gaining weight, you're producing enough milk.

You can tell that your baby is getting enough milk if

- Her nursing is predictable and has the characteristics of a good suck: As she suckles, she opens wide, pauses, and then closes her mouth again.
- She soaks 6 disposable diapers in 24 hours, or wets 8 to 12 cloth diapers. (A disposable diaper feels puffy and heavy when it's soaked.)
- Her stools are mustard-colored, pasty, or watery, with an odor more sweet than foul.

TROUBLESHOOTING

If your infant seems distracted at the breast, he may have nipple confusion (if you use supplementary bottles or a pacifier), or he may be reacting to either an overabundant milk flow or a slowdown in the milk flow.

Some things do affect your milk supply, including birth control pills that contain both progesterone and estrogen, and some decongestants, which are dehydrating.

To improve your supply, these suggestions may help:

- Drink more fluids, especially water. Try to drink an 8-ounce glass of water every 2 hours. Avoid caffeinated teas, coffee, and sodas (check the labels; even cream soda has caffeine), which are dehydrating. (And if you can't do without your coffee or caffeinated soda, drink an equal amount of water to balance it out.)

- Rest, rest, rest. Nap when the baby does. Forget about your housework and other chores; ask, barter, or pay someone else to handle what absolutely must be done—cooking dinner, carpooling older children, etc.
- Allow the baby to nurse as frequently and as long as she wants to, especially during a growth spurt, teething bout, or developmental milestone.
- Take a nursing holiday: a day when you do nothing but nurse the baby all day long, every chance you can, and whenever the baby wants to nurse. Nursing holidays are best spent in bed, on a comfortable couch or recliner, with an ample supply of water and other fluids, and your favorite music, videos, or books on hand. Send the older children to a relative's or friend's house.
- Try dietary and herbal supplements, including fenugreek capsules, blessed thistle tea, fennel seed tea, hops tea, and fenugreek tea (as much as you can drink).

WHEN SUPPLY *IS* A PROBLEM

Most breastfeeding failures are caused by ignorance and mismanagement, but some women are clinically unable to breastfeed exclusively. Among the factors that can compromise milk supply:

- Mothers whose breasts have been surgically enlarged or reduced, especially if the nipple was disturbed or moved.
- Women with asymmetrical or abnormal-looking breasts, whose glandular tissue may be inadequate.
- Mothers of multiples: Even though it is possible to nurse twins or triplets, all the babies must nurse vigorously.
- Premature infant: A premature baby, unlike a full-term baby, often can't empty his mother's breast as effectively as a pump. A preemie's mother usually needs to continue pumping even after the baby is breastfeeding, until

the baby is steadily gaining weight and emptying her breasts by himself

- Babies who fail to gain weight: Infants who are premature, ill, or have a sucking problem, neurological or physical disorder, or are unusually calm often do not feed as frequently as they should, sleeping through feeds that should be every 2 or 3 hours during the first few weeks.

If your baby is not gaining weight appropriately—if she's still under her birth weight after 2 weeks—you need to get professional help immediately. The sooner you resolve your problem, the easier it will be to get your milk supply back on track.

Almost always, education, training, and support can help a mother become successful at breastfeeding. But sometimes lactation problems have medical causes that can't be overcome. Don't feel guilty or bad if you cannot breastfeed for reasons beyond your control. Your baby's health is paramount.

See also Breast Compression; Fenugreek; Finger-Feeding; Herbal Remedies and Supplements, About; Mother's Milk Tea; Overactive Letdown

Supply, Low

Q: I feed my 3-week-old son every 2 to 4 hours, but my milk supply is low. (When I pump, I can only get an ounce.) He seems constantly hungry. What can I do about this?

A: Actually, you're probably not feeding him often enough. A 3-week old baby usually can't go 4 hours between feeds. If his weight is on target, he's alert and gaining well, then the odds are that your supply is adequate. At his age, he's probably going through a growth spurt, which prompts newborns and even settled babies to nurse around the clock.

Is his weight gain on target? (He should be gaining about a half a pound a week, after regaining his birth weight, by now.) Is he producing plenty of wet and poopy diapers? (A 3-week-old baby should produce 8 to 12 wet cloth diapers, or 6 to 8 disposables.) Is he healthy, with good color and firm skin? Is he alert and active, growing in length and head circumference? Newborns typically nurse every 90 minutes to every 3 hours—sometimes more often, so his appetite's on track.

If the answers are yes, your milk supply is fine.

If the answer is no, immediately consult your pediatrician and a lactation consultant. If your milk supply is low, correct the problem now. Your son is at a vulnerable age, and the longer a problem persists, the more difficult it will be to get your breastfeeding relationship back on track.

See also Breast Compression; Diaper Count; Supply Problems, About

Suppositories

See Stools, Infrequent

Surgery and Breastfeeding

Q: I need to have a tubal ligation, but I am not willing to wean my 3-month-old son just for the surgery. Should I be concerned about how anesthesia will affect my breast milk? What about any pain medications I take following the surgery?

A: Many anesthetic drugs are compatible with breastfeeding and are used on moms whose babies are born via c-section, so that they can nurse newborns without problems. Tell your doctor that you're breastfeeding, and ask for anesthesia that's compatible with nursing.

It's a good idea to pump some extra milk for the baby and store it in the freezer or refrigerator for others to give him while you recuperate. (Pump during the nursing sessions you miss.)

One mom who went through gallbladder surgery when her baby was 3 months old found that she could nurse the baby more comfortably by propping a pillow over the bandaged incision. Then she positioned the baby on top of the pillow. The extra padding helps during the first day or so, when the incision area is still tender.

Sushi

Q: Is it OK to eat sushi while you're breastfeeding?

A: Nursing moms can eat most foods, including sushi, that are properly prepared. In Japan, sushi and sashimi (raw fish) is a menu standard, and nursing moms eat sushi there. Only eat sushi prepared by a sushi chef. The main concern with sushi, ceviche, or any other raw fish is that the fish may not be fresh, or that it may come from polluted waters. The biggest danger is toxoplasmosis, which can be contracted by eating raw or undercooked meat.

Sweaty Baby

Q: My 3-month-old has been perspiring a lot during the last couple of days, especially when she's nursing. She sweats so much that her hair gets soaked. I've checked her temperature several times, and it's always normal. She's not too bundled up—it's almost spring—and our heater isn't on. Is this normal?

A: If her temperature and behavior are normal, you probably don't have anything to worry about. (Is she eating, sleeping, pooping, and producing the requisite number of wet—not yellow—diapers daily?) Newborns, as a rule, don't sweat. But as they grow older the sweat glands become more active. If it's warm where you live—or warmer than it's been for a few months—she may be reacting to the seasonal change in temperature.

Switch Nursing

Q: My baby is really sleepy—she nods off before she's even done nursing. My cousin told me to try switch nursing. What's that?

A: Switch nursing can help prevent a baby from prematurely drifting to sleep while she's nursing. All you do is switch breasts as soon as she seems to lose interest in suckling.

When she's no longer swallowing after every one or two sucks, take her off the breast, sit her up, burp her, or change her diaper to wake her up. Then offer the other side. When her nursing slows down again, take her off, rouse her, and go back to the first side.

Keep switching back and forth for 20 minutes or so before you let her go back into a deep sleep. Be certain that she latches on well and takes the breast far back into her mouth as she nurses. Use breast compression to keep her awake long enough to get to the hindmilk in at least one of your breasts—switch nursing can be associated with foremilk/hindmilk imbalances.
See also Breast Compression; Foremilk and Hindmilk; Stools, Green; Sleepy Baby, and Difficult Nursing

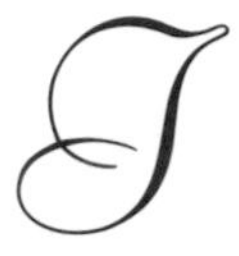

Tail of Spence
See Armpits, Swollen; Breast Lump

Tandem Nursing Newborns
Q: Just how the heck do you get babies to tandem nurse? I get mad and exasperated when I see pictures in books that show peacefully breastfeeding babies as their happy mom cuddles them effortlessly. One of my newborn triplets weighs 6.6 pounds, and he sucks like a Hoover. The smallest one is not quite 4.5 pounds, with such a weak suck that I have to pump to give him a bottle after a feeding. It's impossible to nurse them simultaneously.

A: Tandem nursing does take some practice. (It's a safe bet that the shots of wiggly, crying, or distracted babies were left in the darkroom.)

The first few weeks of nursing newborn twins or other multiples is a challenge. Most moms find it easier to nurse multiples separately at first, because it's so much easier than trying

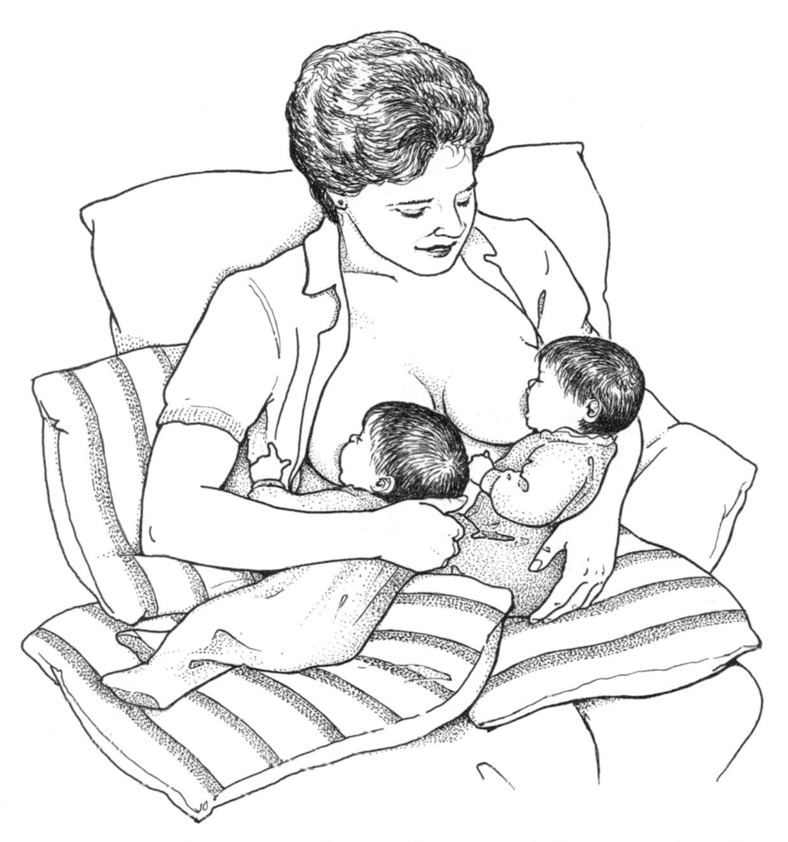

to coordinate them in tandem. Often, one baby is weaker than the other, but the sucking of the stronger baby stimulates the milk flow for the weaker twin. This helps get milk into the weaker baby until that baby's suck strengthens. You may need to supplement the weaker baby if his weight gain and diaper count are not on target.

One mother of twins who breastfed for a year advises: "Just concentrate on getting both the babies nursing reasonably well. Once you get that going, work on doing both of them together. If you look at the pictures of tandem-nursing twins, you'll notice that they are not newborns. Few new infants—twins or singletons—just latch on instinctively and nurse contentedly for 20 minutes."

There are two keys to successful tandem nursing:

First, find a good place to nurse. Forget about the bed. ("Your butt will go to sleep," said one mom.) Most chairs aren't big enough. An oversized armchair or a couch is better.

The second key: Pillows. Lots of them. You'll need one pillow on each side, two crossed across your lap, and a Boppy (a donut-shaped pillow) or a nursing pillow tied around your waist.

Position both babies so they're facing the same direction; it's easier, initially, than the double-football hold. You'll feel as if you're in a fort, but the pillows help keep the babies secure and stabilized. As they get older you'll need fewer pillows, but by then you'll be a pro at this.

Babies old enough to sit straddling your legs are candidates for what one mom calls a "speed feed." The twins sit facing your chest, latch on, and rest their heads in the crook of your arms. (Latch on one first, put his head in the crook of your arm, reach around, and attach the other one.)

Important: With twins, it's easy to get in a rut of letting each one nurse on the same breast. Don't do it. Almost always, one twin has a stronger suck than the other. You'll end up with a plugged duct. Instead, alternate the twins on either breast at every feeding.

See also Positions, About; Twins, Breastfeeding

Tandem Nursing Toddlers

Q: I want to continue nursing my 2-year-old along with my newborn, but nursing sessions turn into wrestling matches. When she sees me with the baby, my daughter fights to get onto my lap and tries to kick or hit the baby. What's the secret to successful tandem nursing?

A: In your case, the answer may be separate nursing sessions. A jealous, wiggly 2-year-old is not a good lap buddy for a newborn who still needs his neck and head supported. Can you breastfeed the baby in a separate room? Another mom's solution was to tell the 2-year-old that their nursing sessions were special private times, when they could be alone together while the baby napped. She also kept a stash of special Big Girl treats—washable glitter pens and paper, stickers, etc.—in the drawer of her nursing station, and doled them out at feeding time. She also found it helpful to allow the 2-year-old to watch *Barney* or *Teletubbies* videos only at nursing time.

Tear Gas, Exposure to

Q: I'm a member of the U.S. Army, and I'm breastfeeding a 5-month-old. Next month, my unit is scheduled for a gas chamber exercise (CS gas). Will CS gas show up in my breast milk after the exercise? If it does, what can I do about it?

A: According to a brochure developed for the Army by a family nurse practitioner, CS gas (orthochlorobenzalmalonitrile—the initials commemorate Ben Carson and Roger Staughton, who first synthesized it) has a relatively short half-life; the same is true of CN (tear gas, chloroacetophenone) and OC (pepper spray, oleoresin capsicium). Breastfeeding women exposed to tear gas during Army exercises—or in other circumstances, as when the Denver woman was inadvertently exposed during a post-Superbowl fracas—should wait 6 to 8 hours before breastfeeding again.

It is critical to wash your skin and clothing thoroughly after being exposed to tear gas. Shower or bathe, and change all your clothing, including underwear, before nursing the baby.

Teething and Nursing

Q: My 5-month-old daughter has already cut her bottom teeth, and now her top teeth are coming in. How can I prevent her from using my nipples to teethe on? She actually leaves little tooth marks on me!

A: You have lots of company—most nursing moms go through the same unnerving experience. Watch for your daughter to become unlatched—she has to break the suction in order to bite—and then slip your finger between her mouth and your nipple.

If she keeps biting, take her off the breast, and tell her again, "No biting!" Even a small baby will get the message.

You might have to repeat this a few times at first, and possibly again when she goes through a teething spell, but she'll learn.

See Biting, About

Teething and Runny Stools

Q: My 7-month-old has two teeth and is cutting another. She's also producing a lot of runny stools—not the mushy, seedy kind, but with mucus. She was exclusively breastfed, but we've started introducing solids. My friend's son is the same age, but he's formula-fed, and he isn't showing these symptoms. Is it teething, or something else?

A: Teething babies do tend to have runny stools and often some accompanying redness in the diaper area. Often, they also poop more frequently than usual—four dirty diapers in a day, for example, instead of one. It's also possible that she is adversely reacting to one of the new foods. Babies are especially prone to dairy and wheat allergies. Do the foods contain any of those ingredients? If the runny stools don't abate after the tooth pops through, or if they increase in frequency and become more like diarrhea, consult your pediatrician.

See also Allergies (Baby's), About

Terms for Nursing

Q: I've heard so many awful stories about older babies yanking at their mother's shirt and demanding "boob" or worse. I'd like to avoid that, but "breast" sounds so clinical. Is there a code word that other breastfeeding moms use for breastfeeding?

A: Families usually evolve their own phrase. When a group of nursing mothers was asked how their babies described breastfeeding, they responded with dozens of terms. Among them: nack-nack, na-na, mook (milk) or Mama mook, T-time, nummies, num-nums, getting the mama. Start using your code word before the baby can talk, so the word you choose is the word your baby uses.

Thirst, Excessive

Q: I'm constantly thirsty. I drink so much water that my friends tease me. I even get up once or twice a night to drink a glass of water. My OB tested me for diabetes, but the results were negative. None of my breastfeeding friends seem to be nearly as thirsty as I am, so what's going on?

A: Don't worry. Most nursing moms, like you, crave water and liquids: 10 8-ounce glasses a day isn't unusual. Drinking plenty of fluids is good for your milk supply, and it ensures that dehydration won't be a problem. Many nursing moms forget to drink enough. That can affect their milk supply and their overall health, especially during hot weather. It's best to drink mostly water, herbal teas, or juice; sodas are loaded with chemicals and caffeine.

Thyroid Scans

Q: My doctor thinks I might have postpartum thyroiditis. She wants me to have a thyroid scan and says I'll have to wean my 2-month-old daughter because the test requires radioactive iodine. But aren't almost all medications compatible with breastfeeding?

A: Thyroid scans are reliable screens for thyroid disorders like postpartum thyroiditis, which is fairly common in the first few months after childbirth. However, your doctor is right: Radioactive iodine must not be given to a nursing mother. It can be found in your milk for weeks after the test and will be concentrated in your baby's thyroid gland.

However, there are alternative ways of treating postpartum

thyroiditis that do not require a thyroid scan. Ask your doctor if it's possible to treat your condition with propranolol or propylthiouracil—two drugs that are compatible with breastfeeding.

Transporting Expressed Milk

See Pumping, About

Thrush, About

Thrush appears as white blisters, as red dots, or as a peeling rash. It is painful for both mother and baby. Yeast is a kind of fungus. Thrush is an overgrowth of yeast. It survives by consuming sugars digested from other sources. Mother and baby must be treated simultaneously. It is extremely contagious; if one of you has thrush, the other almost certainly has it too, or will soon.

Pediatricians or OB/GYNs typically suggest topical ointments, including clotrimazole (in 1 percent or 2 percent concentrations) and Nystatin, which often are used together in treatment. Clotrimazole will work on thrush. If you find the 1 percent cream too slow or ineffective, try the 2 percent miconazole cream. Wash off Clotrimazole before you nurse (use water, not soap), and reapply afterward.

Nystatin prevents the thrush yeast from reproducing; it must be applied to all affected areas four times a day, and you can't nurse for 10 minutes after you use Nystatin. Because it contains sugar, Nystatin can leave your nipples sticky: It never really dries. (If you thought your nipples were sore before, try peeling Nystatin-covered nipples from a nursing bra or nursing pads.)

If you put a little Lotrimin on your nipples, they won't stick to your bra. It's absorbed pretty quickly and thoroughly into the skin. You don't need to wash it off unless your baby wants to nurse the instant you've applied it.

An alternative treatment for thrush is gentian violet. You paint it on your nipples, inside the baby's mouth, on the baby's genitals, and on any other area affected by the thrush. Gentian violet works fast, and it's nearly foolproof, often better at resolving thrush than commercial medications. However, gentian violet has one drawback: Anything it touches will be permanently stained purple. And it takes several days for the gentian violet to work its way through a baby's system or wear off your skin. Plan on wearing dark clothing, using dark towels, and sleeping on dark sheets. On the upside: gentian violet resolves thrush within 2 or 3 days, and you'll have lots of opportunities to teach your baby about the color purple.

Another option for your baby is a relatively new drug called Diflucan, an oral medication that is mixed with water and given to the baby twice a day for 2 weeks. It's a lot easier than swabbing the baby's mouth, and you see results in 48 hours. A pill form of the same medication is an option for adults. One caution about Diflucan: It can damage your liver. Don't take it lightly.

Until the thrush is gone, it's extremely important to sterilize everything that touches the baby's mouth or your nipples. That means boiling all bottle nipples, pacifiers, breast pump parts, and toys. Wash all clothing—yours and the baby's—in hot water. Thrush, as you've learned, is highly contagious.

Don't despair: Thrush can be treated, and you can prevent its return by monitoring your diet and making sure you use breathable, not moisture-proof, nursing pads in your bra. The initial pain should subside within 72 hours.

See also Gentian Violet; Milk Blisters; Nipples, Sore, About

Thrush, Difficulty with Latch-On

Q: My 5-week-old daughter had no problem nursing before she was diagnosed with thrush. Now it's hard for her to latch on—she chews my nipple instead of suckling. What can I do to help her nurse again?

A: A thrush infection can make a baby's mouth sore and itchy, which makes it hard to breastfeed. Even if you're using medications, like Nystatin, the sore, itchy symptoms may take a while to clear up—as much as 72 hours.

Are you being treated for thrush as well? It is extremely contagious, and other family members are susceptible. Make sure you wash your hands frequently, and use disposable towels instead of cloth while you're being treated.

If your baby is gaining weight appropriately, her feeding difficulties are likely to be only temporary. Be careful to pay attention to positioning and latch-on when you're nursing. If she starts chewing your nipple, take her off your breast (slip your finger between her mouth and your nipple). Try again in a few minutes, and bring her in close, so her chin touches your breast as you latch her on. If your breasts still feel full after she nurses, try feeding her again within the hour, or express some milk so you don't get engorged.

Thrush, Recognizing

Q: My right nipple is sore. It has a white blister that appeared a couple days ago, and I'm experiencing shooting pains from the nipple up through the breast. The pains last 10 or 15 seconds, and then stop. It doesn't feel like a plugged duct or mastitis. I thought it might be thrush, but my baby doesn't have a white coating in her mouth. What could it be?

A: It may be thrush—the shooting pains are one symptom. (The classic signs don't always appear at once.)

Does your baby have a bright red rash (red dots, a peeling diaper rash) or seem exceptionally gassy and fussy? Those are other less obvious symptoms of thrush.

See your pediatrician. If it's thrush, you can treat it with an over-the-counter remedy for your baby's mouth and bottom, and your nipples. (*See* Thrush, About.) One way to prevent thrush and prevent reinfection is to be scrupulous about changing your breast pads often—each time you're aware that they're damp—especially if you have an active letdown.

See also Gentian Violet; Milk Blisters; Thrush, About

Time Spent at the Breast

Q: I've heard that babies should nurse for at least 10 minutes per breast at every feeding. My baby sometimes only nurses for 5 minutes, and sometimes for 20 or more. Should I make her nurse longer when she's not on long enough? Take her off when she wants to nurse longer?

A: There's a difference between "being on the breast" and "breastfeeding." If your daughter is actively nursing for 15 or 20 minutes, she may be uninterested in the other breast. If she sucks for only a few minutes and then falls asleep or nibbles, a nursing session can last indefinitely. Your baby will breastfeed best if she's latched on properly, and you can encourage her to nurse actively with breast compression to keep the milk going. She needs to nurse long enough to get the richer hindmilk that provides most of her calories.

Babies usually want to nurse more frequently, and for longer periods of time, during growth spurts. And many babies also nurse for comfort, especially when they're sick or teething. Breastfeeding isn't ruled by the clock: It's a mistake to force a baby to stay on the breast, or to pull off a baby who still wants to nurse.

See also Breast Compression; Foremilk and Hindmilk; Growth Spurts, About; Stools, Green

Toddlers, Weaning

Q: My daughter is 2, and we're usually only nursing at bedtime. She'll nurse a little, then wants to play, and then when she decides she's ready for bed, wants to nurse again. I've been telling her no, which inspires a crying fit, or a tantrum. How can I make weaning less traumatic for both of us?

A: Talk to her about stopping. A 2-year-old wants a sense of control (even if she's not really calling the shots). Ask her how she wants to wean. One mom and her daughter began talking about weaning several months early, agreeing that the daughter's third birthday would signal the end of nursing. Another child came up with a bedtime story cuddle as a replacement. If a 2-year-old doesn't want to give up that nighttime feeding, though, it can be easier to keep nursing until she loses interest.

Sometimes, offering a physical "big kid" substitute like a cyclist's water bottle (with water, not juice or milk) works.

If you're determined to eliminate that nighttime feeding, you must have a partner willing to take over the whole bedtime routine for quite a while.

See also Weaning, About

"Topping Off"

Q: If I normally feed my baby every 2 hours—at 4 P.M. and then at 6 P.M.—but I top him off with a little snack at 5 P.M., when should I feed him again? At his regular 6 P.M. feeding, or at 7 P.M.?

A: The answer depends on your baby, and he can't read a clock. Instead of feeding him on a specific schedule, feed him when he shows signs of hunger. If he seems hungrier than usual, he may be teething or going through a growth spurt.

It's a good idea to feed your baby when he shows signs of being hungry—rooting around, reaching for your breasts—even if it's not "time" to feed him.

See also Feeding Schedules; Schedules for Feeding and Infant Management Programs, About

Traveling by Air with a Breastfed Baby

Q: I'm planning to take my 5-month-old son to Italy—a 50-minute flight, followed by a long 7-hour or 8-hour flight over the ocean, and then another 2-hour flight to our destination. He's mostly breastfed. Got any tips on making breastfeeding easier in a crowded plane?

A: Your baby is at a good traveling age. It's easier to travel with a breastfed baby than a bottle-fed baby—no worries about packing and sterilizing bottles, or bringing enough food. Some tips:

- Takeoff and landing are tough on babies' ears unless

they're nursing or sucking on a pacifier so they're swallowing regularly enough to equalize the pressure on their ears. If your baby won't nurse, try a lollipop or teething biscuit so he'll swallow frequently enough to relieve the pressure in his ears.

- Wear a loose top that you can pull up for nursing.
- Bring bottles for water or expressed milk. If he absolutely refuses a bottle, you'll need to nurse him on takeoff and landing, when his ears will react to the change in air pressure. If he accepts bottles, consider bringing a manual pump, like the Avent Isis, to express milk between flights.
- Bring an extra change of clothes for yourself as well as for the baby, in case of spills or diaper leaks.
- Bring an umbrella stroller or a baby carrier for getting around the airports. If he likes a baby carrier, use that—it's easier to stash, and you can use it for walking down the aisle during flights.
- Make friends with the flight attendants. They can be lifesavers—find you a private (or mostly private) place to nurse, move you to an empty (or emptier) row of seats, and bring water even when the beverage cart is out of commission.
- Take along plenty of "quiet toys" like a busy book and other toys that can capture a baby's interest. If you forget, a glass of ice cubes is a good substitute.

Indispensable: a full container of infant Tylenol, Motrin, or whatever over-the-counter infant painkiller you normally use. If your baby won't nurse during takeoff or landing, give him one dose (as indicated on the directions) about 20 minutes before the plane takes off or lands. And if he gets sick while you're traveling—as many of us do after long plane trips—it will come in handy!

Traveling by Car with a Nursing Baby

Q: We are considering making a long road trip—3 days in either direction, from 8 A.M. to 10 P.M.—so our 4-month-old baby can visit her grandparents. I plan on stopping every 2 hours to nurse. How do babies fare during long drives?

A: Depends on the baby, but usually babies between 2 and 5 months old travel fairly easily—they spend most of the time sleeping. But 14 hours in a car, even with stops every 2 hours, makes for a very long day. Shuffling your schedule to accommodate 4 days of travel each way would make the trip more pleasant for everyone. Here's a sample schedule:

8 A.M. to 10 A.M. Drive

10 A.M. to 10:30 A.M. Stop to nurse, stretch (30 minutes)

10:30 A.M. to 12:30 P.M. Drive

12:30 P.M. to 2:30 P.M. Stop to nurse, eat, stretch (2 hours)

2:30 P.M. to 4:30 P.M. Drive

4:30 P.M. to 5 P.M. Stop to nurse, stretch (30 minutes)

5:30 P.M. to 7 P.M. Drive

7 P.M. Stop for the night

Long drives lull most babies to sleep. If your baby snoozes in the car, schedule your departure for the baby's bedtime or nap time.

Even then, you'll still need to budget extra time for breastfeeding rest stops. It's illegal and dangerous to try to breastfeed and drive simultaneously—or even to unbuckle a baby and nurse her in your arms. Remember that babies tend to alter their eating and sleeping schedules when they're in an unfamiliar place. Bring a blanket, a sheet, and a couple of favorite toys from home, so she'll have objects that smell and feel familiar. Don't be surprised if she wants to nurse more than usual or if she's balky at naptime. Make sure that she gets some time alone (by herself or with you, in a quiet room) to relax from all the excitement and stimulation.

Tube Feeding Lactation Aids

Q: My 10-week-old baby's having trouble gaining weight. My lactation consultant told me to try the Supplemental Nursing System. I'm trying, but I worry that he's confused about how to nurse: He keeps spitting out the tube and my nipple. What should I do?

A: SNS is Medela's trademarked Supplemental Nursing System. SNS and Starter SNS, like other commercial or homemade tube lactation aids, help mothers breastfeed adopted babies, stimulate relactation, and augment a low supply of breast milk.

The baby nurses at the breast from a tube that runs from the mother's nipple to a reservoir of breast milk or formula.

Tube feeding aids seem to work best with young babies, and some babies adapt better to them than others. Babies who are 3 months old or older may have problems with this system, and their newfound dexterity means that they tend to pick at the tubing.

Tube feeding lactation aids help prevent nipple confusion, since the baby nurses at the breast for the supplement as well as for the breast milk. If supplemental feedings are prescribed for a low-weight-gain baby, a tube feeding aid can provide nutritional support while you continue to nurse.

One downside of these aids is that if you want your baby to have only breast milk, you'll be doing an awful lot of pumping. Some moms find themselves pumping every 3 hours around the clock. It can be a lot of work.

Another downside: Tube feeding aids are often incorrectly recommended for babies with a weak suck, breathing/sucking problems, and swallowing difficulties. Some babies have trouble keeping their tongues in position, and push out both the tube and the nipple, and if a baby has a sucking problem, it can be dangerous to force more milk into his mouth. Even when a tube feeding aid is appropriate, sometimes a feeding session can take 45 minutes or longer, followed by another 20 minutes of pumping. By the time you've cleaned the pump parts, it can be feeding time again. On the bright side: Tube feeding aids are meant as short-term solutions, and once you get breastfeeding established, life will be much easier.

If your baby has a weak suck, a lactation consultant or pediatric speech pathologist may be able to help by showing you some exercises and techniques that may help stimulate a stronger sucking reflex. Breastfeeding purists may shake their heads, but if the tube feedings aren't going well, you may be better off bottlefeeding the baby (with expressed milk or formula) and nursing your baby to satisfy his nonnutritive sucking needs.

See also Finger Feeding; Palate, High

Tubal Ligation, Effect on Breastfeeding

Q: My baby is due in about 4 weeks, and I'm planning to breastfeed. I was also thinking of having a tubal ligation done after the delivery. Will this interfere with nursing?

A: Not if you're primarily worried about the medications. Usually, doctors use the same drugs for a c-section as for a tubal ligation. Express your concern to your obstetrician, so she'll be aware that you want breastfeeding-compatible drugs. Your abdomen will be tender for a few days, but not much more than it would have been, anyway, after childbirth. Try some of the nursing positions recommended to mothers who have had c-sections to keep the baby's weight off the incision.

See also Positions, About

Twins, Breastfeeding

Q: I'm a first-time mom, worried about having enough milk to nurse the twins I'm expecting next month. I want to breastfeed them 100 percent. Most of the books say not to worry; supply keeps up with demands. Other moms with twins say that you can't avoid supplementing. Who's right?

A: Usually the other moms. Twins and other multiples are a lot of work, especially for a new mother. Breastfeeding exclusively almost certainly means that you'll be nursing, pumping, and giving supplementary bottles of expressed milk—really a full-time job, especially for the first few weeks. And that's on top of changing their diapers and clothes, and burping and comforting them. It's critical to have full-time help for at least 3 or 4 weeks.

The babies may have a difficult time nursing if they're born before they reach full term. Therefore, it is essential to find a good lactation consultant with lots of experience in working with mothers of multiples.

Plan on renting or buying a breast pump so you can stash some milk. After they're born, make a point of pumping every day after your milk comes in. One mother of twins slept with her sons at night, letting them suckle on and off throughout the night, to maintain her milk supply.

- Call your local La Leche League to ask if there's a multiples group in your area. If there's not, ask if a leader can put you in touch with other breastfeeding mothers of multiples.
- Join Mothers of Multiples or similar support groups in your area for firsthand resources.
- Buy *Having Twins* by Elizabeth Nobel, *Mothering Twins,* by Linda Albi and others, and *Multiple Blessings* by Betty Rothbart.
- Look online for newsgroups like alt.parenting. twins__ triplets for support and advice.

Your goal—100 percent breast milk—is noble, and with plenty of help and support, you can reach that goal. But don't feel guilty if you find that it's necessary to use some formula along with nursing. The twins will still get the antibodies in your breast milk, even if they consume formula as well.

See also Breast Compression; Positions, About; Pumping, About; Tandem Nursing

V

Vaginal Discharge

Q: I've noticed a clear to whitish vaginal discharge lately, even though I haven't resumed my menstrual periods. It's definitely not a yeast infection. I nurse my 9-month-old about 7 times a day. Is this a sign that my periods may be returning?

A: Maybe. Mucus discharges begin about 6 months post partum, or as soon as you regain your fertility, but it could be months before you start menstruating again. It's a good idea to assume that you're fertile again and to use birth control unless you want to get pregnant.

See also Birth Control, About

Vasoconstriction

See Nipple Blanching

Vegetarian Diet

Q: I'm a lacto-ovo-vegetarian: I eat cheese and eggs, but not meat or fish. Will my breast milk be OK for my baby? Should I take supplements?

A: The main concern about a vegetarian nursing mom is whether she's consuming animal protein. If you eat dairy and eggs, you should be fine. Those who don't will want to supplement with vitamin B_{12} and foods fortified with soy milk and fortified yeast. If you don't eat dairy products, you'll need to consume more calcium-rich foods, like leafy green vegetables, tofu, blackstrap molasses, and almonds.

A wide and varied diet is best, even if you're not vegetarian. Try to avoid eating processed foods. Instead, concentrate on legumes, grains, fruits, and vegetables.

Remember that you'll need more calories, protein, and vitamin B_{12} when you're lactating. If you eat too little, your milk supply may diminish. Small frequent meals are the best way to make sure you're eating—and drinking—enough. For specific diet information for vegans and other vegetarians, write to the Vegetarian Resource Group, PO Box 1463, Baltimore, MD 21203; or call 410-366-VEGE; or e-mail vrg@vrg.org

You should be taking a multivitamin to insure that you're getting all the vitamins and supplements you need. If you were anemic during pregnancy, you may need an iron supplement, but otherwise, it's unnecessary—and excess iron can make your baby fussy. Look for supplements that are bioavailable to minimize the side effects.

Vision Correcting Surgery and Breastfeeding

Q: I want to have laser surgery to correct my myopia. I know you're not supposed to get new contacts or glasses when you're pregnant, but does nursing affect your vision too?

A: It can. While you're nursing, your hormones are still in flux, and that can affect the shape of your eye. A responsible eye surgeon will advise you to postpone something as permanent as eye surgery until at least 2 months after you've weaned your baby.

Vitamin B_6

Q: I've heard that large doses of vitamin B_6 can alleviate postpartum depression if you take 100 to 200 milligrams a day. I know I can't use Prozac or St. John's wort, but is vitamin B_6 okay? I'm 3 months post partum, and so depressed I'm nearly always teary or angry.

A: Megadoses of vitamin B_6 are not compatible with breastfeeding. In *Medications and Mothers' Milk,* Tom Hale writes that daily doses of 600 milligrams or more of vitamin B_6 can inhibit the milk supply. He advises against even 100 to 200 mg of vitamin B_6 on the grounds that the biological half-life of pyridoxine (vitamin B_6) is 15 to 20 days in an adult.

People who have taken large doses of vitamin B_6—50 milligrams to 2 grams a day—are more susceptible to seizures and convulsions. Also, large doses have been shown to reduce prolactin production in nursing mothers.

Talk to your doctor about prescription antidepressant drugs. While Prozac is not appropriate for a nursing mother, other antidepressants, including Zoloft and Paxil, are breastfeeding-friendly.

See also Antidepressants and Breastfeeding

Vitamin K

Q: My aunt told me that formula has more vitamin K in it than breast milk does and that formula-fed babies are less likely to have hemorrhages than breastfed babies. Is this true? I thought breastfeeding was better in every way than formula.

A: Formula does have a higher concentration of phylloquinone—vitamin K—than breast milk does. However, according to a recent study, a nursing mother can increase her baby's phylloquinone intake by taking vitamin K supplements. You can reduce the risk of hemorrhagic disease in an exclusively breastfed infant by making sure that she receives an injection of phylloquinone at birth and that you take a supplement of vitamin K (5 milligrams daily) for the first 12 weeks after birth.

Vomiting Baby and Breastfeeding

Q: My 7-month-old baby has some kind of tummy bug and throws up a lot. It seems kind of pointless to keep breastfeeding. Should I stop breastfeeding her until she's well again?

A: No. The best medicine for a baby's gut infection is breast milk. Except under extraordinary circumstances—when a baby is so dehydrated that she must be hospitalized, for example—breast milk supplies the only food and fluid she needs. Stop the solid foods until she's recovered, but keep nursing her. It will comfort her and will keep her hydrated better than any artificial rehydrating solutions can. Even if she's vomiting, a small amount of breast milk will be absorbed. Try nursing her in the bathtub when her illness is at its worst.

If the vomiting continues longer than 24 hours, or if she shows signs of dehydration, see your pediatrician immediately.

See also Dehydration; Reflux, or Spit-Up?

W

Warming Refrigerated or Frozen Expressed Milk

Q: Is there a quick way to warm refrigerated milk? My husband ends up with a squalling baby in one arm and holding the cold bottle under a warm faucet. By the time he gives her the milk, he's frazzled, and she's so upset that she won't take the bottle. And she refuses to take cold milk.

A: Try heating the cold bottles in a large pot or jug of hot water. It will still take 15 to 20 minutes to warm a bottle straight from the fridge. Never microwave breast milk—it kills the nutrients and heats the milk so hot that it will burn a baby's tender mouth.

Forethought helps. Your husband should start the warming process before the baby starts showing the obvious signs of hunger—rooting, sucking her fist, fussing. If 2 hours or so have passed since her last feed, it's probably a good idea to warm up a new bottle.

If she's still reluctant to take the bottle, try different nipples. Many moms have success with Avent.

See also Bottles, About; Pumping, About

Water Supplements

Q: My mother desperately wants to feed my 2-week-old daughter. I want the baby to have breast milk only. She sneaked the baby a bottle of water yesterday when I was showering, and I hit the roof. I worry about nipple confusion. She says the baby needs extra water because it's so hot. The weather is very warm. Should I let my mom give the baby water?

A: Feeding water to newborns is neither necessary nor recommended by pediatricians. Water is nutritionally empty, and even in hot weather, the baby doesn't need it. Your breast milk contains enough water to keep her well hydrated. (She may want to nurse more frequently during warm weather; let her.)

A study of 1,677 mothers and babies found that giving newborns supplementary water can actually be dangerous. A 2-week-old infant like yours—or any other infant under 5 weeks old—is susceptible to oral water intoxication if given too much water. The sodium in her bloodstream becomes so diluted that the baby's body can't function normally. This can lead to abnormally low body temperatures, bloating, disorientation, and in extreme cases seizures.

Older babies—6 months and up—can have small amounts of supplementary water or diluted juice (one third juice to two thirds water). Still, breast milk provides the best nutrition throughout a baby's first year of life. It's nutritionally dense, is readily available, and is the most complete food, calorie for calorie, you can offer.

It's likely that your mother really wants the sense of closeness with her new grandchild, so suggest an alternative. Perhaps when you're finished nursing, your mom would be willing to burp the baby. Or she may enjoy rocking the baby to sleep (or while she sleeps, if the baby falls asleep at your breast).

See also Dehydration; Diaper Count; Hot Weather and Nursing

"Watery" Milk

Q: My expressed breast milk looks too thin, like skim milk, especially when I compare it with formula. I've been eating lightly to lose my pregnancy fat, but should I start eating more fatty foods?

A: Mature breast milk does look thinner than formula, but that doesn't mean that your milk is "too watery." Expressed breast milk, left to stand (even refrigerated or frozen) will separate, with the fat rising to the top. Human milk contains all the nutrients your baby needs. It is so easily absorbed that breastfed infants need less breast milk, ounce for ounce, than formula. The fat content of your milk changes throughout a single feeding, starting with the thinner foremilk, followed by the higher-fat hindmilk. Foremilk is about 2 percent fat; hindmilk consists of 10 percent fat (sometimes more).

You should eat a well-balanced diet to maintain your energy and your milk supply. But eating more high-fat foods will not make your milk creamier.

Weaning, About

You thought it was tough to establish breastfeeding? Brace yourself for weaning! It's usually long, slow, and wearing physically and emotionally.

Gradual weaning is best for you and for your baby. Dropping only one feeding every week or so means that you'll be less susceptible to engorged breasts and possible inflammation. It's easier on the baby, too—less stressful and traumatic. Before you start, stock up on nursing pads—many women leak when they're weaning—and don't plan on wearing silk blouses or anything else that stains easily. Loose shirts and big button-front vests or cardigan sweaters are good camouflage when you're weaning.

Start by eliminating one feeding session, and then, after a week or so, dropping another one. If your baby is especially reluctant to wean, you may need to drop one feeding session in 48 hours (rather than one feed in 24 hours). It may take longer to wean, but it will be easier on both of you.

For the first cut, choose a feeding session that can be bypassed as painlessly as possible. Most babies want to hang onto the nursing sessions associated with bedtime—the day's first feeding, naptime feeding, and bedtime.

You can eliminate some feedings without completely weaning if you'd prefer not to go cold turkey just yet. You can usually keep one or two nursing sessions a day, even after cutting out the rest.

If you do want to totally wean, and your baby is under a year old, you'll need to find a brand of formula that your baby will take. If you have a friend whose baby uses formula, ask for a couple of tablespoons' worth, and see if your baby likes it. If you don't know any formula users, buy the smallest unit on the shelf—it's cheaper to buy formula in bulk, but it's a waste of powder and money if your baby doesn't like that brand.

When you begin dropping nursing sessions, replace that time with another kind of cuddling or special time. Instead of regarding weaning as something to deny your child, think of it as a time to expand your child's horizons by offering new tastes and foods and customs. Instead of hurrying the process, let it take its own pace, and the transition will be easier on you both.

There's more to breastfeeding than nutrition: It represents love, comfort, trust, attachment. Try keeping a stack of picture books near the rocker, so you can find a new use together for a favorite chair. It's a good idea to cuddle in a position that's different from the one you typically used for nursing—e.g., holding your child facing away from your chest as you read a picture book together, or balancing her on your feet or legs to play airplane.

Don't be surprised if your baby, unprompted, starts ignoring customary nursing sessions once you've begun weaning. Many babies and toddlers self-wean. Your little one may nurse twice one day, and once the next, and want to nurse twice again the day after that. She may give you her signal that she wants to nurse, but then squirm off your lap as you start to pull up your shirt.

You may notice that you're feeling discouraged, sad, or distracted during the weaning period. It's not unusual to be a little depressed. Your body is going through hormonal changes again. Weaning can be painful, physically and psychologically. After all, this is one sign that your baby is growing up and that you won't always be the center of his universe. Try collaborating on a memento of this time together by making palm prints or footprints—yours alongside his.

The flavor of your milk will change as you wean. It may taste salty or even a little sour.

It may take a while for your milk to dry up. It's not unusual to continue lactating for several months or more than a year after weaning.

See also Engorged Breasts; Galactorrhea; Leaking, About; Nursing Strike

Wean, Pressure to

Q: My son has breastfed for 6 months, and my mother-in-law is nudging me to wean him. She says I've nursed longer than most moms and implies that there's something weird about wanting to continue nursing him. I'd prefer to nurse him until he weans himself. What can I say to get her off my back?

A: Tell her, matter-of-factly, that the American Academy of Pediatrics recommends breastfeeding for at least the first year of a child's life, and that the World Health Organization encourages moms to breastfeed even longer. (And remember—when your mother-in-law raised her children, the prevailing philosophy may have been different from that of today.)

No matter how old your baby is, each time he nurses, he will receive benefits, including antibodies. The AAP studies found that breastfed babies are less colicky, are better-nourished, are more resistant to infections and illnesses, and thrive better than formula-fed babies.

And if you want some tacit support from your baby, there are T-shirts (in baby and toddler sizes) printed with messages like "Don't Ask Me When I Am Going To Wean" and "Got Milk?" Your local La Leche League chapter members can suggest stores or mail-order catalogues that offer the shirts.

See Appendix

Weaning Readiness

Q: My 11-month-old son went from nursing 10 times a day to four or five times in 24 hours, sometimes less. For the last couple of weeks, he seems more interested in "talking" and playing than in nursing. He gains well but has never been a long nurser—3 to 6 minutes per side, and he was done. Now that he's eating solid foods (three meals, plus a couple of snacks) he's only nursing three times a day: at dawn, after his afternoon nap, and before bed. Is he weaning himself? If not, how will I know when he's ready to wean?

A: Not necessarily. As babies get older they become more efficient nursers, taking what they want quickly. They're also more interested in playing and exploring. Have you noticed an increase in night nursing? If he nurses more at night, he's making up for any calories he doesn't get during the day. Has he started eating more solid foods? That can reduce the amount he nurses, especially if he's eating a lot of solids.

If he seems uninterested or less interested in nursing, no matter what time it is, he may be beginning to self-wean. Do you have to do what one mom calls "the baring the breast dance" to start a nursing session? Since he's still nursing, apparently with no problems, and is gaining well, relax. He may be weaning himself—and for some babies, it's a slow process. (Bonus for you: The gradual cutback on nursing sessions will mean you'll have an easier time during weaning.)

See also Weaning, About

Weaning to Cup

Q: I've breastfed my daughter, 5 months old, exclusively. Now I have to wean her, and she won't take a bottle. Well, she'll take it, but only to play with the nipple. She won't drink from it. Can I just wean her straight to a cup? How?

A: How about trying a sippy cup instead of a bottle? A 5-month-old who's never had a bottle is likely to have strong negative feelings about artificial nipples. But a sippy cup doesn't mimic anything she knows, and she may see it as an interesting challenge.

Look for spillproof sippy cups. Even newborns can drink surprisingly well from cups.

Weaning: Reluctant Toddler

Q: My son, 2-1/2 years old, doesn't want to wean, but I'm ready to stop. I've tried to go cold turkey without success. His screams are intolerable (and they only prompt letdowns, so it's pointless to let him cry). He also won't go for the "big boy" pep talks or for bribes. Do you have any suggestions?

A: Does your son have certain nursing sessions that he prefers? Does he tend to nurse himself to sleep at night, or first thing in the morning—the two times that many toddlers like best?

Try cutting down just one session at a time. (Don't forget: Nobody understands "no" better than a toddler.) You'll need to decide how many nursing sessions you're willing to tolerate. (Some moms can handle one or two nursings a day, but not four or five.) To successfully eliminate one nursing session, you'll need a lot of help from your partner. If you're dropping a prenap nursing session, start by adding something to the routine, like your partner reading a story after you nurse. After the story time becomes part of the routine, let your partner begin the routine alone, or gradually shorten the amount of time you nurse. His favorite nursing session should be the last to go. And if he wakes up at night and wants to nurse, your partner will have to be the one to respond to his cries.

See also Weaning, About

Weaning Tips

- Change the routine. Have Dad take over the bedtime or nursing-time tasks that Mom formerly handled (dressing, reading stories).
- Take the weaning child for a long car ride at nursing time.

- Introduce a "transition object"—a toy, lullaby tape or book, for example—at 12 to 15 months, so the baby learns to associate something besides nursing with going to sleep. This will make it much easier to wean your baby.
- Offer a snack—juice and a favorite food—at nursing time.
- The favorite nursing sessions (e.g., morning and bedtime) should be last to go.
- Manage engorged breasts with a "bra salad"—raw cabbage leaves tucked between your breast and the bra.
- Manually express as much milk as you can when you feel painfully full.
- Sleep in a stretchy exercise bra, with nursing pads to soak up leaking milk. It's not unusual to leak for more than a month after weaning. Some women's breasts still produce a drop or two of milk more than a year after they wean their baby.

Weight Loss

Q: I know that when you're breastfeeding, you need more calories, but I'd really like to drop my pregnancy baby fat. I try not to eat too much, but I can't seem to lose weight. Is it because I'm breastfeeding?

A: Not necessarily. Women who've never nursed their babies also have trouble returning to their prepregnancy size.

Although some women can lose or maintain their weight when they're breastfeeding, many women find it tough.

Don't plunge into a diet the day you come home from the hospital. The first 6 weeks or so are hectic enough without counting calories. Most obstetricians advise against dieting during that period, anyway, when your body is adjusting to childbirth, and your uterus is going through involution—tightening up and eliminating lochia.

It's pretty common to have a hearty appetite when you're lactating. Some women are almost constantly hungry. If that's your case, no wonder you're having trouble shedding some pounds.

A lactating woman burns an extra 200 calories daily. That's not much—the caloric equivalent of a large baked potato or a couple of cookies. If you're eating approximately 1,800 calories a day and doing some sort of aerobic exercise at least three times a week your body may not be ready to lose weight yet.

Two studies conducted in the 1980s concluded that breastfeeding alone doesn't guarantee weight loss, and another study in 1991 found that 22 percent of breastfeeding mothers actually gain weight. Weight loss and lactation is an area that hasn't been researched extensively, but generally, weight loss is most difficult for older women and for women who have gained more than the recommended amount of weight during pregnancy.

If you're eating more than about 1,800 calories a day, or if those calories are mostly empty (fat and sugar), you'll have to adjust your diet.

Go heavy on greens and grains, light on fats and meat, and lighter on treats. It's hard to be as active as you were before the baby was born, but you'll need to step up your activity level. Walking is good exercise, and with a stroller or a front- or back-carrier, it's reasonably baby friendly. Try exercising in the morning, when you're more likely to consistently fit a workout into your schedule and before naps, chores, and general chaos chew up your time. If you exercise aerobically between five and seven times a week, your metabolism will respond, and you'll start losing weight.

If you need an extra push, Weight Watchers has a nursing mother's diet that many moms recommend enthusiastically.

Another helpful resource is Ellen Behen's *Eat Well, Lose Weight While Breastfeeding*. The author is a dietitian and mother who knows firsthand about breastfeeding.

Remember: Don't try to lose too much too fast. Weight loss, like weaning, is likelier to be successful if you do it gradually. On average, a mother takes about 5-1/2 months to return to her prepregnancy weight.

Weight, Appropriate for Babies

Q: My 11-month-old baby is hitting all the developmental milestones on target, except that after he was about 6 months old, he stopped gaining as much weight as he should according to the growth charts. He weighs only 17 pounds—he hasn't doubled his birth weight (9 pounds, 8 ounces). Should I be worried about his eating habits?

A: Actually, he sounds as if he's pretty much on target—he's only a bit below doubling his birth weight, and he still has a month to go. And he was a big newborn.

Also, remember that scales vary, and sometimes a baby's weight is incorrectly recorded.

For breastfed babies, standard pediatric growth charts function as a reference rather than an inflexible diagnostic ruler. Standard growth charts are based on formula-fed infants, whose growth patterns differ measurably from breastfed babies.

Generally, breastfed babies tend to be chubbier and longer than formula-fed babies during the first 6 months, as measured by the growth charts. It's not unusual for a breastfed baby to be in the 90th percentile for weight and/or length during that period. Many parents panic that their babies are growing too fast, worry that the babies are getting fat, and restrict nursing sessions to try to control their weight. (This is a mistake: Your baby will be hungry, and your breasts, reacting to the lower demand, will stop making as much milk as your baby needs.) At 4 months, a healthy breastfed baby may look like an infant Buddha, but the story often changes 2 months later.

The cliché about older breastfed babies is that they're long and lean. Once they reach 6 months, their growth slows down—compared with formula-fed babies' growth—and levels off or falls to the 50th percentile or lower. A breastfed baby who's 7 months old may be in the 20th percentile according to the growth charts but still is perfectly healthy and normal. A pediatrician unfamiliar with the growth pattern characteristic of breastfed babies may recommend unnecessary supplements of formula, or even weaning.

See also Nursing Constantly; Weight and Growth Charts, About

Weight Gain and Newborns

Q: I breastfeed my 3-week-old whenever he wants to nurse. He's gained about 1-1/2 pounds since birth. My pediatrician is concerned that he's gaining too fast and wants me to limit feedings to every 4 hours or so. I tried, but I can't stand hearing him cry. He wants to breastfeed more often than ever. Is it possible for a breastfed baby to gain too much weight so fast?

A: Not really. Most newborns are expected to gain about half a pound a week, although since many babies lose a little weight during their first week, they may not hit that target as dependably as your son did.

Your son's increased hunger may be a sign that he's hit his first growth spurt, when some babies seem to nurse constantly. Denying him the chance to nurse on demand not only deprives him of the milk he needs to get through this spurt but may decrease your own ability to produce as much milk as he needs. Ask for a second opinion if you want to continue breastfeeding.

See also Growth Spurts, About; Nursing Constantly; Weight and Growth Charts, About

Weight and Growth Charts, About

Most pediatricians use the National Center for Health Statistics (NCHS) growth curves as a reference for measuring a baby's height and weight. The NCHS growth chart for children under age 2 is based largely on the Fels Longitudinal Study, which was conducted from 1929 to 1975 in Yellow Springs, Ohio. The Fels Study reflects the growth of infants and toddlers whose diet consisted primarily of infant formula, supplemented with solids (rice cereal, pureed fruits) often introduced when the babies were 4 months old or less. The weights of babies in the Fels Study were skewed to the heavy side. (Many of the Fels babies had a tendency toward childhood obesity.)

Many pediatricians, lactation consultants, and others are concerned that the NCHS growth chart, because it's based on formula-fed babies, is inappropriate for breastfed babies.

Pediatricians who strictly follow the NCHS growth chart may misdiagnose a healthy breastfed baby as being underweight. They may advise mothers that their milk is inadequate, and recommend supplementing (or replacing) breastfeeding with formula and introducing baby cereal and pureed foods.

Breastfeeding proponents, including the World Health Organization and the World Health Assembly, have recommended replacing the current growth chart with a reference that is based on healthy breastfed babies. A WHO committee recommended that the new chart include a larger population sample from several countries, and further recommended using the new chart as a screening tool—diagnosing failure to thrive or obesity—rather than as a self-contained diagnostic tool.

Weight Gain, Slow

Q: Should I be concerned about my daughter's weight gain? She weighed 7 pounds, 10 ounces at birth. Now she's 8 months old and weighs about 13-1/2 pounds. My doctor is concerned that she's not gaining enough weight, even though she nurses 3 or 4 times a night and eats 3 jars of baby food a day.

A: Some babies are slow to gain weight. The weight charts used at pediatricians' offices are based on formula-fed babies. Several studies have shown that breastfed babies don't follow the same growth curve—their growth and weight gain starts tapering off, relative to the charts' growth curve, at about 6 months.

Part of the reason for your baby's relatively slow weight gain could be her increasing level of activity. She's crawling, cruising, and starting to be interested in pulling herself up. As long as she is producing enough wet and poopy diapers, is alert, and has energy, she's probably fine. A baby is supposed to double its birth weight at the first year, and she's got a few months to go.

Is your doctor aware that she's primarily breastfed? Is he aware that breastfed and formula-fed babies tend to grow at different rates? (Remember, the cliché is that breastfed babies are long and lean.)

Ask your doctor if she's being weighed on the same scale each time you take her to the office. Different scales can read heavy or light.

Ask your doctor about her growth and weight gain relative to her parents' size and physique. (Does your family, or your husband's, sway toward the small and light?)

And consider the bright side: Small babies use small diapers, which have more to the package, for the same price, as larger-size diapers.

See also Weight and Growth Charts, About

White Spot on Nipple

Q: I have a white spot about the size of a blackhead on my nipple. It won't respond to warm compresses, different nursing positions, or anything else. I tried to pick it off with a pin, but that hurt. And it reappeared anyway. What is it? How can I get rid of it?

A: Not by popping it—but you learned that the hard way! Several problems present as white spots. You could have a milk blister, a clogged pore, or the first sign of thrush.

If it is a clogged pore in the nipple skin, it's a nuisance cosmetically, but otherwise it won't interfere with breastfeeding. Clogged pores are common, especially if you pump frequently. (The solution: Set the pump to a lower intensity.) One mom who pumped exclusively—she couldn't breastfeed, but was determined to give her baby breast milk—reported that the skin on her nipples was white, like dead or scarred skin, until she stopped pumping. Even then, it was more than a month before her nipples regained their normal coloring.

You should also check the symptoms of plugged ducts and thrush. Both can be serious problems if you fail to get medical attention.

See also Milk Blisters; Plugged Ducts, About; Thrush, About

Witches' Milk

Q: My newborn son's breasts are swollen, and yesterday they leaked something that looked like milk. Is this normal?

A: Yes, it's normal, even in boys. Many babies are born with swollen breast and genital buds, the result of glands and ducts stimulated by their mother's pregnancy hormones. Newborns, girls and boys, may secrete drops of milk during the first few days after birth. The folk name for these secretions is "witches' milk." The secretions should stop within the first week.

Work and Breastfeeding

Q: I'm a nurse practitioner who pumps in the office I share with a (female) co-worker who gripes that my pump is noisy and claims that my milk presents a health hazard! She told our supervisor that I should wear disposable gloves and that I should pump in the restroom. How can I handle this?

A: She sounds like a difficult co-worker. Can you arrange another meeting with your supervisor? Tell him about the U.S. Surgeon General's Healthy People 2000 Goal of increasing the number of women who attempt to nurse their newborns, as well as increasing the number of mothers who persevere with breastfeeding instead of turning to formula. (You can get a copy of the policy statement from the La Leche League or from the Internet; *see* Appendix.) There also is proposed legislation, bolstered by research showing that employees who breastfeed have less absenteeism from infant illness, to give employers a tax break if they give lactating employees a 1-hour break to express milk.

Explain diplomatically to your supervisor that it's inappropriate to use the restroom for pumping when, in essence, you're preparing your infant's meals. Is there a small, private area, separate from your office (apart from the restroom) where you can pump?

If your supervisor is concerned about your co-worker's claims, inform him that although breast milk is a body fluid, latex gloves are not required for handling it. The virus that causes HIV and

AIDS is as fragile as it is lethal, and it cannot survive outside the body for more than a few minutes.

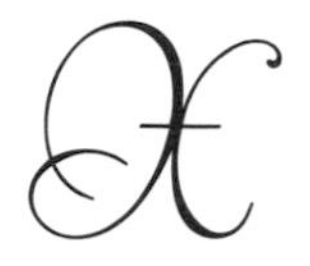

X-Rays, Chest

Q: I'm nursing my 8-month-old, and I'm due for a chest X-ray, as well as a mammogram. Are X-rays compatible with breastfeeding?

A: According to the American Academy of Pediatrics' committee on drugs, X-rays do not have an adverse effect on breast milk. You can go ahead with your chest X-ray as long as no radioactive isotope is used.

However, it's possible that the radiologist may want you to wait for the mammogram until after you've weaned the baby. Mammograms are harder to read when a woman is lactating, although it can be done. If you do get a mammogram, don't be surprised if your breasts leak a little milk when the technician positions the plates. Even after weaning, it takes only a little pressure to coax a little milk or colostrum from once-lactating breasts.

Other imaging methods, including MRI scans and CT scans, do not affect your milk.

One exception: Thyroid scans, which require you to take radioactive iodine, are not recommended for breastfeeding mothers. However, there are alternatives to this test. Ask your doctor about them.

See also Thyroid Scans

X-Rays, Dental

Q: Now that my daughter is 3 months old, I need to go to the dentist for some work I couldn't have done while I was pregnant. Should I be worried about X-rays, since I'm still nursing? Could my milk be affected somehow?

A: No, dental X-rays don't have any effect on your milk. The lead shields are meant to prevent damage to possible pregnancies. However, if it eases your mind, you can ask your dentist to use two lead shields, as an extra buffer. So go ahead and make an appointment with the dentist.

Y

Yeast Infection, Oral

See Thrush, About

Yeast Infection, *Candida*

Q: My obstetrician diagnosed a *Candida* infection in my nipples and milk ducts. He told me to try gentian violet, which I thought you were supposed to use for thrush. What's the difference between *Candida* and thrush?

A: Nothing, really. Basically, we're talking about yeast infections here. Some doctors believe that yeast infections are especially prevalent because antibiotics are so widely and readily used that *Candida albicans,* the harmless version that normally cohabits peacefully on our bodies, becomes more overgrown than an Arizona suburb.

Infection sets in when the skin or mucous membrane is broken down—when your nipples are cracked or sore, for example. The oozing that accompanies cracked nipples transforms *Candida albicans* into its nasty alter ego.

If you have a yeast infection, it's a good idea to assume that your baby does, too. (Or vice versa: If your baby's mouth is covered with thrush, you probably have it too, even if you're symptom free.)

See also Thrush, About

Yeast Infection, Vaginal

Q: I have a yeast infection, and I need to treat it. But I don't want to stop breastfeeding my 7-month-old. The medication instructions say that it's not safe for nursing moms, and when I asked my doctor about it, he was sort of wishy-washy, leaning toward weaning. Can you help?

A: If your yeast infection is vaginal, and you're using an over-the-counter medication such as Monistat, you don't need to wean. Nonprescription antifungal medications leach only negligible amounts into breast milk. Even Diflucan, a prescription antifungal, routinely is prescribed for breastfeeding mothers fighting thrush and other *Candida* infections.

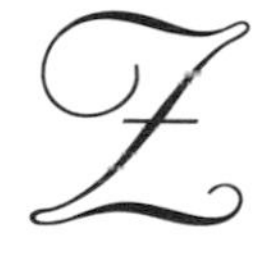

Zombie Mommy

Q: My 7-month-old daughter never has slept for more than 2 hours straight at night. When she wakes, I have to nurse her back to sleep, or she wails at full throat. It's gotten worse in the last 2 weeks. She wakes every 20 to 45 minutes after one or two 2-hour stretches. We've ruled out an ear infection, and we're sleeping in a family bed so I can nurse her without getting up. What else can we do?

A: Is she nursing vigorously because she's hungry, or sucking half-heartedly until she falls asleep again? If she's not gulping and swallowing, she may be nursing for comfort or because she relies on sucking to put herself back to sleep. If that's the case, this is a sleeping problem, not a nursing problem, and you'll need to help her find other ways of calming herself enough to sleep. (Rubbing her back or giving her a favorite lovey may help.)

Could she be teething? Is she drooling more than usual, or gnawing on toys, or sucking more for comfort than for milk? Try using a teething gel or a widely available homeopathic remedy, like Hyland's Teething Tablets, to relieve the pain. If that works, you'll know her problem is teething. And if not, at least that rules out teething as a problem.

Many babies are wakeful at significant milestones—learning to sit up, crawl, pull up, etc. They typically return to their old sleeping patterns within a couple of weeks, so if that's what is causing your daughter's nocturnal energy, the end is in sight.

It's hard never to get more than 2 consecutive hours of sleep, but this too shall pass. Another mom got through the wakeful spells by reminding herself of that saying that intelligent babies sleep less. It worked for her.

See also Teething and Nursing; Appendix

Appendix: RESOURCES

BOOKS

Mamatoto: A Celebration of Birth by Carroll Dunham and the Body Shop (Viking)

The Complete Book of Breastfeeding by Marvin S. Eiger and Sally Wendkos Olds (Workman)

Medications and Mother's Milk by Thomas W. Hale (Pharmasoft Medical Publishing)

The Nursing Mother's Companion by Kathleen Huggins (Harvard Common Press)

Breastfeeding Your Baby by Sheila Kitzinger (Knopf)

The Womanly Art of Breastfeeding by the La Leche League International (Plume)

Breastfeeding and the Working Mother by Diane Mason et al. (St. Martin's Press)

The Breastfeeding Answer Book by Nancy Mohrbacher (La Leche League)

Dr. Mom's Guide to Breastfeeding by Marianne Neifert (Plume)

Breastfeeding Your Baby: A Practical Guide For the New Mother by the Nursing Mother Council of the Boston Association for Childbirth Education (Avery Publishing Group)

So THAT'S What They're For! by Janet Tamaro (Workman)

The Fussy Baby: How to Bring Out the Best in Your High-Needs Child by William Sears (La Leche League International)

VIDEOS

"Breastfeeding Your Baby—A Mother's Guide: Positioning" #610V010 (English); 800-435-8316

Excellent Medela video includes a good demonstration of the football hold, and superior instructions for the classic breastfeeding positions, plus advice. May be available at larger La Leche League lending libraries.

"Guide to Successful Breastfeeding" with Jane Morton; VHS.

Practical tips from a physician. May be available at La Leche League lending libraries.

"Breastfeeding: A Special Relationship" VHS in Spanish.

TOLL-FREE INFORMATION AND BREASTFEEDING PRODUCTS

Ameda/Egnell (Hollister) breast shells, breast milk freezer bags: (800) 323-4060

International Academy of Compounding Pharmacists (for a local compounding pharmacist to provide advice about medications): (800) 927-4227

La Leche League: 800-LA LECHE (800) 525-3243

Medela, Inc. (baby scales, breast milk freezer bags, breast pumps, breast shells, lanolin, Supplemental Nursing System): (800) 435-8316

Mommy's Little Helpers: (800) 859-3559

The National Association of Postpartum Care Services: (800) 45-DOULA

Nurture Parenting Products (Yummy Mummy nursing clothing): (888) 301-2266

INTERNET

American Academy of Pediatrics: <http://www.aap.org>—Information on breastfeeding, pediatric medicine and related issues.

Ask the Doctor/Maternal & Child Forum: <http://www.medhelp.org>—Nurses and doctors from Detroit's Henry Ford System answer breast feeding and child care questions.

Breastfeeding Mothers' Support Group: <http://www.members.tripod.com/~bmsg/>. Based in Singapore, with advice relevant for moms everywhere.

Breastfeeding advice group: <http://www.parentsplace.com/cgi-bin/objects/lactation/bf164.data>—Articles and information about breastfeeding problems and questions.

Breastfeeding advice: <http://www.onelist.com/subscribe.cgi/breastfeeding>

Breastfeeding- and Baby-Friendly hospital list certified by the World Health Organization: <http://www.aboutus.com/a100/bfusa/hospital.htm>

Breastfeeding information, advice, and link to World Health Organization growth chart for breastfed babies: <http://www.clark.net/pub/activist/bfpage>

Breastfeeding information, articles, activism: <http://www.ProMoM.org> (Promotion of Mother's Milk)

Breastfeeding information, articles, parenting advice:<http://www.compleatmother.com>

Formula recall weekly advisory: <http://www.fda.gov/opacom/hpnews.html>

Herbal milk-boosters and other lactation aids: <http://www.breastfeedinghelp.com>

Human milk bank information: <http://www.leron-line.com/milkbank.htm> Information about milk banks in the United States.

LactNet library: <http://library.ummed.edu/archives/lactnet.html>—Articles and information about breastfeeding, lactating, medicine and breastfeeding, other issues.

La Leche League: <www.lalecheleague.org>—La Leche League's Web page.

Medical advice about breast inflammations/infections, etc.: <www.obgyn.net>

Newsgroups: alt.support.breastfeeding, and misc.kids.breastfeeding. (Search Usenet or DejaNews to locate.) Helpful, lively newsgroups with many links, practical advice and debate about relevant issues from moms and some lactation consultants who keep up with the newsgroup.

Nursing bra resources

Motherwear—<http://www.motherwear.com>

Trevas—<http://www.trevas.com>

Extra Emphasis—<http://home.earthlink.net/~arizon aarobextrae.html>

<www.ElizabethLee.com>

Nurture Parenting Products: <www.nurture-parenting.com>

Parenting advice links: <www.eyeontheweb.com>

Pumping advice: <e-mail pump@interlink-bbs.com>

Pumping advice, frequently asked questions: <www.enscript.com/pump/FAQ>

Starting solid foods: <http://www/parentsplace.com/cgi-bin/boards/startingsolids>

Tandem nursing (twins, triplets)

alt.parenting.twins-triplets

<www.nurturing.ca/tandemnursing.htm>

SPECIAL NEEDS

Breastfeeding the Adopted Baby by Debra Peterson

Breastfeeding the Infant with Special Needs by Donnal Dowling, et al. (March of Dimes Nursing Modules available online)

Breastfeeding the Premature Baby by Jack Newman, M.D.; <www.bflrc.com/newman/overheads>

"Newborns Who Need Special Care," World Health Organization paper: <www.who.int/chd/publications>

MILK BANKS

Human Milk Banking Association of North America, PO Box 370464, West Hartford, CT 06137-0464; (860) 232-8809; e-mail lahmbana@tiac.net

Mothers' Milk Bank, Valley Medical Center, 751 South Bascom, San Jose, CA 95128; (408) 998-4550

Mother's Milk Bank, Women's Hospital, Columbia-Presbyterian St. Luke's Hospital, 601 E. 19th Ave., Denver, CO 80218; (303) 869-1888

Wilmington Mothers' Milk Bank, Medical Center of Delaware, PO Box 1665, Wilmington, DE 19579; (302) 733-2340

Community Human Milk Bank, Georgetown University Medical Center, 3800 Reservoir Rd NW, Washington, DC 20007; (202) 784-6455

Human Milk Bank, Central Baptist Hospital, 1740 S. Limestone, Lexington, KY 40503; (606) 275-6502

Memorial Health Care Regional Milk Bank, 119 Belmont St., Worcester, MA 01605; (508) 793-6005

British Columbia Children's Hospital Milk Bank, 4480 Oak St., Vancouver, BC V6H 3V4, Canada; (604) 875-2345, ext. 7607

Triangle Lactation Center and Milk Bank, Wake Medical Center, 3000 New Bern Ave., Raleigh, NC 27610; (919) 250-8599

NURSING BRAS, MAIL ORDER

Cameo Coutures, Dallas, TX: (214) 631-4860. Custom-made nursing bras.

Extra Emphasis, PO Box 1725, Tahoe City, CA 96145; (916) 581-0848 (information); or (800) 539-0030 (orders only). Specializes in hard-to-fit clients; special bras have large bands, large cups, and small bands, small cups.

Motherwear, PO Box 114, Northampton, MA 01061-0114; (413) 586-7532 or (800) 950-2500. Nursing bras to 48H, nursing shirts, etc., up to 3X, plus other baby and nursing products.

BREAST PUMP MANUFACTURERS (RENTAL)

Ameda Egnell (distributed by Holister, Inc., in the US), 20000 Hollister Dr., Libertyville, IL 60048-3781; (800) 323-4060; http://www.hollister.com

Medela, Inc., P.O. Box 660, McHenry, IL 60050-0660; (800) 835-5968; http://www.medela.com

SUPPORT ORGANIZATIONS

Breastfeeding National Network, Medela, Inc. PO Box 660, McHenry, IL 60050-0660; (800) 835-5968

Cleft Line (referrals to local cleft palate/lip support groups), 1829 E. Franklin St., Suite 1022, Chapel Hill, NC 27514; (800) 242-5338

Doulas of North America, 1100 23rd Ave. E., Seattle, WA 98112; (206) 324-5440

International Childbirth Education Association, PO Box 20048, Minneapolis, MN 55420-0028; (612) 854-8660

International Lactation Consultant Association, 4101 Lake Boone Trail, Suite 201, Raleigh, NC 27607; (919) 787-5181

La Leche League,1400 N. Meacham Rd., Schaumburg, IL 60173-4048; 1-800-LA LECHE

Lamaze International, 1200 19th St. NW, Washington, DC 20036-2401; (800) 368-4404

National Association of Postpartum Care Services (doula information); (800) 453-6852

National Down Syndrome Congress, 1605 Chantilly Dr., Suite 250, Atlanta, GA 30324-2369; (800) 232-6372

National Organization of Mothers of Twins Clubs, Inc. (and other multiples clubs), PO Box 23188, Albuquerque, NM 87192-1188; (800) 243-2276

Nursing Mothers Council National Office, PO Box 50063, Palo Alto, CA 94303; (650) 599-3669

Special Supplemental Nutrition Program for Women, Infants and Children (WIC): Contact your local or state health department for the nearest clinic serving eligible clients

The Tandem Nursing Support Association, c/o Nurturing Magazine, #373, 918 16th Ave. NW, Calgary, Alberta, Canada T2M OK3

Index